The Medical Interview: A Primer for Students of the Art

The Medical Interview: A Primer for Students of the Art

JOHN L. COULEHAN, M.D., M.P.H., F.A.C.P.
Associate Professor of Community Medicine
Associate Professor of Medicine
University of Pittsburgh School of Medicine
Pittsburgh, Pennsylvania

MARIAN R. BLOCK, M.D., A.B.F.P.
Assistant Professor of Community Medicine
Chief, Division of Family Medicine
University of Pittsburgh School of Medicine
Pittsburgh, Pennsylvania

ESSENTIALS OF MEDICAL EDUCATION SERIES

DAVID T. LOWENTHAL, M.D., Ph.D. / Editor-in-Chief
Professor of Geriatric Medicine and Adult Development
Professor of Medicine and Pharmacology
Mount Sinai School of Medicine
New York, New York

F. A. DAVIS COMPANY • Philadelphia

Library of Congress Cataloging-in-Publication Data

Coulehan, John, 1943-
   The medical interview.

   Bibliography: p.
   Includes index.
   1. Medical history taking. I. Block, Marian, 1947-   II. Title. [DNLM: 1. Medical History Taking. 2. Physician-Patient Relations. WB 290 C855m]
RC65.C68 1986 616.07′51   86-6382
ISBN 0-8036-1995-2

Authorization to photocopy items for internal or personal use, or the internal or personal use of specific clients, is granted by F. A. Davis Company for users registered with the Copyright Clearance Center (CCC) Transactional Reporting Service, provided that the fee of $.10 per copy is paid directly to CCC, 27 Congress St., Salem, MA 01970. For those organizations that have been granted a photocopy license by CCC, a separate system of payment has been arranged. The fee code for users of the Transactional Reporting Service is: 8036-1995/87 0 + $.10.

To Our Families

ESSENTIALS OF MEDICAL EDUCATION SERIES

Editor's Commentary

To Our Students

This series has been developed to help you review essential biomedical facts and concepts and reinforce basic clinical skills. Because medical science is forever evolving and expanding, you should expect to spend a lifetime building upon a knowledge base gained through your required curriculum. It is our hope that these texts, together with your educational program and faculty support, will help you develop patterns of independent learning and skills of analytical thinking and clinical decision making. Therefore, in many of the volumes, our authors further aim to challenge you with questions and problems similar to those you will experience in classroom and clinical situations as well as in national examinations.

Although a large component of your education will be devoted to scientific theory and technologic principles, we believe that you must not lose sight of the importance of your patient as an individual. Accordingly, we have tried to maintain a humanistic focus where applicable in both the basic science and the more clinical texts in this series.

In this volume, Drs. Coulehan and Block introduce you to the art of the medical interview—an art that can be learned best by practicing specific skills. They believe that medical interviewing and doctor-patient interactions are at the core of medicine and therefore should be central in medical education as well. *The Medical Interview: A Primer for Students of the Art* is designed to be a guide for students who are just learning to take a medical history as well as for those who, as clinical clerks, are beginning to have sustained contact with patients. Although the authors deal primarily with basic history taking, the skills that are the subject of this book serve as building blocks for all doctor-patient interactions and are thus the essence of the "art" of medicine.

DAVID T. LOWENTHAL, M.D., Ph.D.
EDITOR-IN-CHIEF

vii

Foreword
From the Patient's Perspective

This splendid book is both interesting and important because it is concerned with real patients in the natural setting of clinical medicine. Given that the work of medicine is about the care of real patients, it is strange but true that this book is one of the few of its kind.

The fact of this volume's distinctiveness requires some comment. Solid grounds exist for considering the 20th century as the period when science entered medicine in full force. The contributions of science to medicine pervade every dimension of clinical medicine, from understandings of basic mechanisms of disease, to the discernment of diagnostic technology, to the power of current therapeutics.

Another trend characteristic of 20th century medicine is the emphasis on the sick person—the subject of medical care. How the illness interferes with the patient's function claims our attention not only for its diagnostic information but also because of our genuine concern for the interference in the patient's life caused by the disease. Treatment choices are commonly made with the patient's viewpoint in mind.

Another aspect of the pre-eminence of the person in medicine is the current understanding that how a disease presents itself, what course it runs, and what its outcome will be depends in part on *who* the patient is. We see diseases as confined to organ systems or parts of the body, whereas the cumulative effects of disease on the person extend, we know, to the person's relationships with others, to the family, and even, on occasion, to the community.

From the late 19th century and well into the early decades of this century, physicians were not directly concerned with patients' perspectives. They were almost solely interested in finding what disease a patient had. That attitude is natural enough considering the fact that diseases as they are presently known had just been "invented" in the early years of the 19th century and were *the* exciting advance of the times. The two fundamental tenets of classical disease theory are that each disease is characterized by a unique pathologic abnormality and that every disease has a unique cause. Little wonder that physicians spent their time trying to ferret out the pathologic abnormality that was the seat of the patient's illness, as well as hunting for its particular cause. In the light of these beliefs, it is not surprising that there was not much room in medicine for the sick person *as sick person.*

On March 19, 1927, Francis Peabody published in the *Journal of the American Medical Association* a now-famous paper called "The Care of the Patient," in which he pointed out the detrimental effect on patient care that is produced by the single-minded pursuit of disease. He showed the problems raised when a patient is dismissed as having nothing wrong just because no disease can be found to account for the symptoms. The startling feature of his essay, and what makes it a landmark, is that it discusses these issues *from the point of view of the patient.* Peabody was not alone, however, in promoting the importance of the sick person in medicine. The blossoming of the modern discipline of psychology and the work of Freud and his followers were also of great importance in promoting an appreciation of the effect of emotions in the production and amelioration of illness. Since the Second World War, the place of the subject in medicine—the importance of the sick person—has become an established part of the medical scene.

Or has it? A multitude of external evidence supports the idea of the central position of the sick person. Entering medical students are imbued with the importance of the patient. Virtually every medical school curriculum has courses devoted to humanities in medicine, ethics, or similar person-oriented subjects. In sharp contrast, however, is the perspective one gets from within a modern teaching hospital, where it is clear that the central place of the sick person is more an ephemeral ideal than a reality. In the wards of academic centers, students and house officers are rewarded for their command of science and technology rather than their understanding of the perspective of the patient. How can it be that something as characteristic of the medicine of this era as the centrality of the sick person is so *informally* accepted and so formally problematic? The answer lies in the almost paradoxical fact that *both* the importance of the sick person *and* science are what characterize modern medicine. It is in exploring the contest and friction between science and personal values that we will see what an important book Drs. Coulehan and Block have written.

Acceptable knowledge, from a scientific point of view, is objective, reproducible, and predictable. Numeric data seem best to meet the ideal, but other artifacts such as roentgenograms, electrocardiograms, spirometric tracings, and slides of tissue are also acceptable. In medicine, we call such information "hard" data. On the other hand, information that is subjective, value-laden, or which cannot be measured is considered unscientific and believed to be of lesser value. It is often called "soft." Medical scientists believe that soft data should be replaced by hard data at all times. Unfortunately, the knowledge and information by which we come to know the viewpoint of the sick person—bodily feelings, emotions, needs, desires, fears, beliefs, future concerns, lived past, relationships, and so on—are *always* "soft," subjective (in that they have to do with a subject), value-laden, and unmeasurable. *It has always been so, it will always be so, and it cannot be otherwise.*

The truth of the previous sentence has not been easy for medicine, doctors, or science to accept. Instead, three solutions to the quandary posed by the unscientific nature of personal information have been tried. One has been to banish the person from medicine as practiced. In this view, doctors take care of diseases, and personal factors are thought to be, at best, matters of sentiment and at worst, contaminants that impede the diagnosis and treatment of disease. This has merely led to bad medicine in which technologic imperatives rule over human needs—we do things because they can be done rather than because they should be done.

A second solution has been to try to *force* personal information into the mold of the scientific ideal by creating questionnaires and scales that can be handled numerically. This may have some uses, but for the care of individual patients it is worse than useless—worse because it fools the doctor and puts off the inevitable recognition that personal information *cannot* meet the scientific ideal.

The third commonly attempted solution is to live by a double standard. On the one hand, formal recognition is given to scientific knowledge and information, while pretending that nothing else is really important in medicine. At the same time, the importance of the perspective of the sick person is given informal acknowledgment by valuing highly such things as caring, humaneness, or compassion, which are thought to be the characteristics of a good doctor. Double standards require people to say one thing but do another. They are inherently unworkable.

Personal information does not meet scientific standards; this cannot be denied. There is another way out of the quandary, however, that is better than the three described. Accept the fact that certain standards of information (scientific) apply to certain types of knowledge—the objective facts of nature. Other standards of information apply to the other type of knowledge—personal information about sick persons. It is not that one is better, the other worse; they are inherently different. A scientist's personal feelings about how RNA transcription occurs, for example, are useless information. Numeric measurements of the patient's feelings are equally useless. The real questions are not whether information is scientific or not, or which type is better; the real questions for doctors are: What is the problem? What kind of information do I need to solve the problem? How do I get the information? How do I ensure maximum reliability of information? How do I think about it? and How do I apply it?

The importance of this book lies in its direct address of these questions. The volume takes the information that patients have to offer about their diseases and themselves to be of fundamental importance in the care of sick persons. The book then offers methods for getting at that information through the relationship between doctor and patient. Then it provides ways to think about and use the information that is developed through the interaction of the doctor with the patient.

The volume's distinctiveness arises from the manner in which its subject is approached. Its teachings are systematic, its system based on theoretic principles, which the authors make perfectly clear. The reader is free to agree or disagree with the theory. But because theoretic underpinnings are provided, readers do not have to model themselves after the authors in order to make effective use of the teachings. This is a refreshing change after all the interviewing cookbooks!

One thing more. I hope that this book will stimulate readers to take part in the development of methods of thinking about the personal information obtained from patients, methods of inquiry that will be as powerful for this type of information as are scientific methods for the objective facts of nature. This book is a wonderful way to begin to learn the ideas and skills that doctors employ throughout their lives—the same ideas and skills that are the first step toward the advances in methods of thought that are necessary to continued progress in medicine.

ERIC J. CASSELL, M.D., F.A.C.P.
New York, New York

Preface

Our course in medical interviewing and ultimately this book originated from our perception of a paradox. We found, on the one hand, that most faculty members in our university emphasized the importance of history taking, both in their lectures to students and house staff and in their discussions of individual patient cases. Certainly, in their own medical practices they valued the clinical art of interviewing. On the other hand, medical school and residency curricula put very little emphasis on the systematic teaching of history taking or medical interviewing. Our medical students received a "little black book" that outlined a patient history and gave a long series of suggested information to obtain. The seeming contradiction between the avowed value of history taking in patient care and its neglect in the curriculum troubled us. There was a sense that students should "pick up" interviewing skills through experience; yet there were few opportunities to monitor or direct that experience. As students and residents discussed clinical problems on rounds, it seemed apparent that historic data tended to be valued considerably less in the decision-making process than other, more "scientific" data.

The central purpose of this book is to demonstrate that good interviewing skills are not simply a matter of being nice to patients or of attending to psychosocial issues; good interviewing skills allow the doctor to obtain more complete and more accurate data about the illness, data that contribute to better diagnostic and therapeutic decisions. These skills also facilitate written communication, leading to more effective case descriptions. Good doctor-patient communication is not simply pleasant or desirable, it is at the core of the science and logic of clinical medicine. Good communication leads to the further benefits of more cost-effective medical care and fewer malpractice claims.

But just what are the specific interviewing skills and how can one teach them? We went to the literature to learn how others had observed and taught medical interviewing and then went to our own practices, and to those of some of our peers and residents, to learn more about the process of interaction between doctor and patient. We did this by audiotaping and videotaping many interviews, listening to the tapes, watching them, transcribing them, and studying them. We found many good interviews, some bad ones, and a number of patterns. We observed, in the best history taking, a dynamic balance between an open-ended, nondirective approach that promoted patient acceptance, rapport, and willingness to tell the story, and a clear, task-oriented structure that directed the interview toward accurate and precise information.

We developed a course for second-year medical students based on these convictions and the data we had acquired. The course contributed to our experience; it refined our conclusions, particularly about how best to *communicate* the skills of communication. We found that a micro-skill approach, developed by Carkhuff, Ivey and Authier, and others for counseling situations, could be adapted to teaching history taking. Yet we were careful that the emphasis on process be used to improve one's precision and accuracy in obtaining data and not be confused with counseling *per se*. This book developed over a period of years from materials we prepared for students in the medical history taking course. However, the finished product is not tied to a specific format or method of teaching. Our objective here is to provide a step-by-step approach to the practice of medical interviewing—one that can be useful to students and house officers who simply read the book, try out its methods, and reflect upon their experiences, as well as being useful to those who employ it in the context of organized instruction.

The book includes numerous examples of doctor-patient interactions. The large majority of these are abstracted from real taped interviews, although in every case we have removed any personal references that might serve to identify the doctor or patient. In a few cases we have taken the liberty to alter (mostly by shortening) the transcripts in ways that serve to demonstrate specific points more compactly. We wish to thank the patients and physicians who permitted us to tape and study their interviews, providing a rich resource for understanding and teaching the skills of history taking.

Some may feel that there are certain things missing from a book of this nature. We have deliberately not included a chapter on the written history (or "write-up"), as the requirements for this vary from institution to institution. We also struggled with the hazy border between the history and the physical examination and decided not to include a section on the mental status examination. Although the method used for formal evaluation of mental status is part of the interview, we believe this is more a part of the physical examination in the sense of detecting signs as opposed to symptoms.

We are grateful for the inspiration and assistance we had from many persons in preparing this book. First, we want to acknowledge two outstanding physician-educators whose influence pervades this text. Eric J. Cassell, M.D., taught us how to observe the doctor-patient interaction *systematically* and supported us throughout this endeavor; his remarkable insights, based on the analysis of thousands of taped interviews, have culminated in the recent two-volume work *Talking with Patients*. Alvan Feinstein, M.D., first taught us that the medical history is a basic source of scientific data about the patient and his or her illness and made us aspire to find the science in the art of history taking. His ideas permeate the text and are derived from his extraordinary course "Introduction to Clinical Medicine" at Yale and his book *Clinical Judgment*.

Faculty members of the medical interviewing course at the University of Pittsburgh have provided fruitful ideas, thoughtful discussion, constructive criticism, and unwavering support through the years. We would like specifically to acknowledge the efforts of Lili Penkower, Noelle Poncelet, Laurel Milberg, Donna Nardini, and Joel Merenstein. Penna Drew read the entire manuscript in draft stage and gave valuable suggestions and encouragement. Larry Pacoe spent hours reviewing tapes with us, teaching us to uncover hidden meanings. Many colleagues shared their insights about the personal meaning of illness to patients; in particular, Lee Bass taught us about the difference between "actual" and "ostensible" reasons for seeking care. Kenneth Rogers, our department chairman, was supportive and ran interference for us throughout this project. Finally, we express our thanks to Judy Smith, who not only put up with the administrative nightmare of coordinating students, classrooms, and faculty for several years but also prepared this manuscript through its many revisions.

Although each of us had primary responsibility for writing certain chapters and for selecting and editing transcripts, this book is a joint product; in a very special sense it is a truly collaborative effort, and we are both responsible for the entire text.

JOHN L. COULEHAN, M.D., M.P.H., F.A.C.P.
MARIAN R. BLOCK, M.D., A.B.F.P.

Contents

Time after time I have gone out into my office in the evening feeling as if I couldn't keep my eyes open a moment longer. . . . But once I saw the patient all that would disappear. In a flash the details of the case would begin to formulate themselves into a recognizable outline, the diagnosis would unravel itself, or would refuse to make itself plain, and the hunt was on. Along with that, the patient himself would shape up into something that called for attention, his peculiarities, her reticences or candors. And though I might be attracted or repelled, the professional attitude which every physician must call on would steady me and dictate the terms on which I was to proceed.

William Carlos Williams, from *The Autobiography,* reprinted in W. C. Williams, *The Doctor Stories.* New Directions, New York, 1984.

Introduction: The Poor Historian

History-taking, the most clinically sophisticated procedure of medicine, is an extraordinary investigative technique: in few other forms of scientific research does the observed object talk.

Alvan Feinstein, *Clinical Judgment*

They cluster in the hall on rounds, eight of them—students, house officers, and the attending physician—creating turbulence, obstructing flow. A medication nurse pushes her cabinet around them on the way down the hall, while the breakfast lorry closes in from the other direction. The intern begins his presentation: "Mr. Blank is a 52-year-old man who presents with abdominal pain . . . the patient is a poor historian . . ."

The attending physician learns that this sick person "claims" to have a number of symptoms and that he is "apparently" taking several medications. The intern hastens to add that the patient's compliance is poor, he doesn't seem to understand his illness, and he is, after all, a "poor historian." Having dispensed with the preliminaries, the intern moves on to reporting the patient's physical findings and initial laboratory data. At this point he drops all qualifiers: the magnesium level does not **seem** to be 2.2, it **is** 2.2. The attending physician lets that phrase "poor historian" roll around inside his head, perhaps because of his unconscionable lack of interest in magnesium. The matrix of numbers vibrating among the house officers and students takes on a life of its own, while he wonders about the patient's poorness. He knows what the intern is trying to tell the group with the phrase "poor historian." The intern does not mean that the man is an impoverished professor of history. Nor does he mean the patient is a failing history student. No, he is saying in precise medical shorthand, "I was unable to reconstruct a logical story of the illness in my conversation with this patient. We did not communicate well." Reflecting further, the

1

attending physician finds the term "poor historian" acceptable but wonders if the attribution is correct. Perhaps the intern would be more correct in saying, "The history is unclear because I'm a poor historian."

This vignette illustrates how data we obtain from speaking with the patient and the therapy we accomplish through the process of doctor-patient communication are not often topics for discussion during medical rounds. While we consider information about serum magnesium a fit topic for discussion, its accuracy and precision assumed, knowledge about the precise pattern of symptoms or the patient's beliefs about the symptoms appears less scientific and less relevant. The third-year medical student soon learns to spend less time listening to the patient and more time among his peers at the nurse's station agonizing over the meaning of a magnesium value. We accept responsibility for how well we perform a bone marrow, interpret an x-ray, or insert a proctoscope. We rarely blame the patient for a poor marrow, yet we believe the hospital is full of patients who perpetrate poor histories.

These attitudes—attitudes that permeate medical education—are based on two premises. **First,** "objective data are more important than subjective data, numbers are more important than words." There is a belief that the subjective data—what the patient tells us—is necessarily lacking in quantification and so it must also be lacking in scientific value. In other words, what patients feel, the suffering they experience, and the disability and pain that haunt them, which they can describe only indirectly with words, are secondary to those physiologic quantities that can be observed directly by physicians. Physicians address what they believe **causes** all this suffering and pain: altered physiology, abnormal biochemical findings, disease. If you correct the bad numbers, the suffering will go away. The person and the illness are subjective; the disease and the numbers generated by machines are objective.

The second premise is that the art of doctor-patient communication is something "you will pick up as you go along." While you must study biochemistry, pharmacology, and gynecology in a systematic manner, you need not study human behavior and the art of medicine. Unlike "science," understanding persons and acquiring skill in communicating simply come to you with experience. This belief follows from the first: if subjective data are of secondary importance, the method of obtaining such data is not a major factor in medical education.

This book about medical interviewing is based on radically different premises. We hold that the person and illness are primary, and only through a careful understanding of the person's experience of illness can we discover the diagnosis and choose the most effective and efficient therapy. Moreover, the "subjective" can often be considerably more "objective"—more precise, accurate, and useful—than the laboratory tests and procedures we consider so scientific. Far from being on the periphery of medical education, we believe that medical interviewing and doctor-patient interactions are at the core of medicine and should be central in medical education.

This book is about interviewing medical and surgical patients, persons suffering from physical illness. Skill in talking with patients is not an art reserved for psychiatrists. In practice, primary physicians spend the largest part of their clinical time talking with patients; they generate most of their diagnostic hypotheses on the basis of the history; and a large majority of the significant bits of information they use arise from this dialogue. Experienced clinicians claim that, in general, about 70 percent of diagnoses are made on the basis of patient interviews and over 90 percent on the basis of history and physical examination (Cutler, 1979). The medical interview and the physical examination, which is a continuation of the same doctor-patient interaction using different techniques, are basic skills of medical practice. In both cases, you use yourself and your words or actions as instruments to gain information. You also use yourself as a mode of therapy through talking with patients. This is what the English psychiatrist Michael Balint meant when he taught that the "doctor is the drug" (Balint, 1972). Just as your stethoscope is the instrument of auscultation of the heart, you are the instrument of the medical history. Just as you study to gain skill in getting the most out of your stethoscope, you must study to gain skill in getting the most out of your verbal interaction with the patient.

In the last 30 years, many investigators have looked at the process of interviewing and have analyzed individual components of that process. It has become clear that while interviewing and the doctor-patient relationship are parts of the "art" of medicine, it is an art that can be learned best by practicing specific skills. Good history taking is not a matter of common sense, nor does it depend solely on an extensive knowledge of pathophysiology, nor does it come necessarily with experience. It is a skill that can be broken down into its component parts, and it can be learned. That is the subject of this book.

Medical interviewing is a basic clinical skill. This book is addressed primarily to first- and second-year medical students, students who are about to begin their professional interaction with patients. It is designed to be a guide for those who are just learning to take a medical history, as well as a resource for those, a little further along in their education, who are beginning to have some sustained contact with patients as clinical clerks. Our particular emphasis will be on the micro-skills of the initial patient interview. Although we will deal extensively with basic history taking, the same skills serve as building-blocks for all types of doctor-patient interactions. They are at the core of the "art" of medicine.

The first chapter introduces you to the concept that history taking can produce accurate and precise information. You can apply some of the same "objective" standards to interviewing as are applied to the serum magnesium measurement in our hospital vignette. The next chapter presents certain qualities—empathy, respect, and genuineness—and demonstrates with many case examples that the physician can make these operational to promote good verbal and nonverbal communication. Subsequent chapters then take up the various components of a medical history, in each case separating out and illustrating specific skills pertinent to that part of the interview. We then consider the "difficult" patient and difficult situations that often arise when we take care of the "ordinary" patient. In the last part of the book, we illustrate the doctor's total influence on the patient through a model of the healing act, which has focal, behavioral, and symbolic components. You begin to influence your patient even as you take the medical history and do the physical examination. The final two chapters apply our model to demonstrate how your skill influences patient compliance, behavior, anxiety, and suffering.

CHAPTER 1

Art and Measurement: History Taking as a Clinical Skill

> The means of testing, required to give an inferential element any claim whatsoever to be *knowledge* instead of conjecture, are the data provided by observation—and *only* by observation.
>
> John Dewey, *Propositions, Warranted Assertibility, and Truth.*

Biomedicine is based on a group of theoretical sciences. Clinical medicine, however, is a practical science: it is a science of helping ill people get well, rather than a science of understanding disease. As with any other science, clinical medicine has basic units of observation, basic quantities of measurement, and basic instruments for obtaining these measurements. The basic units of observation are signs and symptoms, the quantities of measurement are words and sometimes numbers, and the instrument for obtaining most of these measurements is the medical practitioner (Feinstein, 1967). Like any other scientific instrument, the clinician must be as objective, precise, sensitive, specific, and reproducible as possible in making observations about the patient's illness.

OBJECTIVITY

What does it mean to be objective in interviewing a patient and taking a medical history? **Objectivity** means removing one's own beliefs, prejudices, and preconceptions before making observations; it involves removing **bias** or systematic distortion from one's observations. Other words for objectivity are accuracy and validity. Your observations should correspond to what the patient really felt and experienced. If, for example, you start out by expecting a typical history of a certain illness and discard things the patient says that do not seem to fit, you are not being objective. Consider this interview taken from Platt and McMath (1979), in which the physician "knew" the patient had severe lung disease and so was unable to hear or follow up on the chief complaint:

Dr: Hello, I'm Dr. X; are you Mrs. Y?
Pt: Yes, I'm glad to know you.
Dr: What sorts of troubles have you been having?
Pt: I've been going downhill for two years. Nothing seems to be working right.
Dr: What is the worst part?
Pt: My legs. I have constant pain in my legs. It's gotten so bad I can't sleep.
Dr: What about your breathing?
Pt: Oh, that's all right. I can breathe fine. I just hurt so bad in my legs.
Dr: Are you still smoking?
Pt: Yes, with this pain I've gone back to cigarettes for relief. But I'm down to a half a pack or so a day.
Dr: Are you having pains in your chest?
Pt: No.
Dr: How about cough?
Pt: No, I hardly ever cough.
Dr: How much are you actually able to do?
Pt: Well, I was able to do everything until about two years ago, but now I can hardly walk half a block.
Dr: Why is that?
Pt: My legs. They hurt.
Dr: Do they swell up?
Pt: Well, they've been a bit swollen the last two or three weeks, but the pain is there whether they swell or not.
Dr: All right, I want to ask you some things about your medical history now.

The physician in this case seems to ignore the patient's leg pain; when she complains about it he replies with questions about breathing. He is undervaluing certain kinds of information—ignoring what he does not expect—while overvaluing others, data related to a diagnosis that he "knows." This not only is unscientific and could lead to a missed diagnosis, but also it is highly likely to make the patient feel ignored. When patients feel ignored they tend to say less and less, and data vital to making the diagnosis may be lost.

This is how the same physician might respond on a better day:

Dr: Hello, I'm Dr. X; are you Mrs. Y?
Pt: Yes, I'm glad to know you.

> Dr: What sorts of troubles have you been having?
>
> Pt: I've been going downhill for two years. Nothing seems to be working right.
>
> Dr: What is the worst part?
>
> Pt: My legs. I have constant pain in my legs. It's gotten so bad I can't sleep.
>
> Dr: Pain in your legs. Tell me more about that.
>
> Pt: Well, it's gotten so bad I can hardly walk half a block.
>
> Dr: You mean the pain forces you to stop?
>
> Pt: Yes, that's exactly it. And, well, it gets better when I stop, but it never really goes away. Even at night when I'm lying still it wakes me up, it's so bad.

The patient here is giving a history consistent with severe peripheral vascular disease, a story the physician is now attending to. The patient is now able to volunteer important details about the leg pain that not only aid the diagnostic process but also help her feel understood. The skill in being objective requires first effective listening and then effective feedback to the patient of what you have heard; in other words, you let the patient know that you hear what she is saying.

Interpretation versus Observation

It is easy to confuse **interpretation** with **observation.** Medical students are sometimes encouraged by preceptors and house officers to use terms that are really interpretations as opposed to descriptions of actual or primary data. One example of such a term is "angina," which means a certain kind of chest pain due to coronary artery disease. This is an interpretation implying a specific etiology. The primary data of the symptom might be something like "substernal discomfort of a dull, pressing nature, lasting about three minutes, brought on by exertion and relieved by rest." The use of terms such as "angina" is a method of shorthand necessary for quick thinking and talking in medicine; such shorthand terms are often interpretations of data and are fine to use when the symptom has indeed been shown to be, in this case, secondary to coronary artery disease. **But** if you interpret the symptom prematurely, you may lose the data that point to the correct diagnosis. Premature interpretation compromises objectivity.

This is an example of a 68-year-old woman who lived for several years with the diagnosis of angina (that is, coronary artery disease) because her physician did not listen for primary data. Here is how she described her chest pain:

> Dr: Tell me about this chest pain.
>
> Pt: It's a soreness in here, right through here *(pointing to mid-chest)*

> a lot. Some pain in my arm and a feeling in here. And a burning in the middle here and a burning in my throat.
>
> Dr: When does this seem to come on?
>
> Pt: Oh, it can be anytime, doctor. Sometimes I even get it in the middle of the night.
>
> Dr: How about when you walk or are active in any way?
>
> Pt: No, I can just be sitting.

Despite the fact that the patient did not have exertional pain relieved by rest, she had a complete cardiac work-up including coronary angiography; even though all tests proved negative, she carried a diagnosis of "coronary artery disease." Finally, a new physician heard the "burning" and the nocturnal occurrence of pain and ordered an esophagograph and upper GI series; the physician discovered massive esophageal reflux and spasm. Perhaps it would have been more serious to overlook coronary artery disease, but for the patient much was lost: frightened that she might drop dead at any moment of a heart attack, she persisted in her belief that she had heart disease and was unable to be rehabilitated to an active life.

Objectivity means not only separating your own interpretations from the data but also separating the patient's interpretations from the data. This is important to remember when a patient tells you "My ulcer is acting up," or "My heart is giving me a lot of trouble," or "I'm here for my Hodgkin's disease." In such instances, the patient is interpreting certain data, or symptoms, to mean an ulcer or heart disease or is reporting a diagnosis instead of the primary data. This is an example of a 78-year-old man who called his physician with the following complaint:

> Pt: I don't know what's wrong. Somebody said I must have had the flu but it's lasted so long and I've tried everything and I don't know what to eat, so I just had to call and find out what you thought because it's been going on now two weeks and you know me, I don't call unless I really have to. And someone said I must have appendicitis or what's that thing that old people get?

The patient here focuses on the etiology of his problem and does not present data about his symptoms. All we know is that, whatever has been going on, it has been going on for about two weeks. The physician's next response might be:

> Dr: Well, some people who get the flu do feel sick for quite some time.

While this shows that the physician has heard the patient's theory, the physician still would not know what is going on. A better response might be:

> Dr: Well, some people who get the flu do feel sick for quite a while, but I'm not sure you had the flu. What exactly were your symptoms?
>
> Pt: Well, I had severe diarrhea—just like water—for a few days and I hurt low down in my belly. And weak, awful weak.

The doctor now has some primary data with which to start putting the diagnostic puzzle together. Although the patient's interpretation should be separated from primary data, the interpretation should not be ignored; it is important to acknowledge the belief as legitimate whether or not you agree with it and to accept it as necessary to managing the patient when the time comes to explain the rationale for a particular therapy or course of action.

PRECISION

Precision is a second characteristic of a scientific instrument or measurement, which refers to how widely observations are scattered around the "real" value. Here, we are dealing not with a systematic bias that leads purposefully in one direction or another, but rather with the random, unsystematic error, induced by vagueness, poor listening, or lack of attention to detail. In taking a medical history, the basic units of measurement are words; words are used to describe sensations perceived by the patient and communicated to the physician. Words are verbal measurements and should be understood precisely; they must, therefore, be as detailed as necessary and as unambiguous as possible. For example, if a patient complains that he is tired, does that mean he gets short of breath on exertion, that his muscles feel weak, that he lacks the desire for physical activity, or that he is sleepy? Although the physician may correctly perceive that the patient says he is tired, the physician may have no idea what is actually being described unless he or she gains enough detail to distinguish among dyspnea on exertion, muscle weakness, and somnolence. In order to do this, the next question might go something like, "What do you mean by 'tired?' " or "Does this tiredness keep you from doing anything?" The good interviewer finds out with as much precision as possible what the patient is actually experiencing. The following is an example of a physician trying to get as much detail as possible about a chief complaint of headache:

> Dr: What do you mean by "migraine headaches?"
>
> Pt: The last two headaches—I had two headaches last week, one on Monday and one on Thursday. Now they weren't real, real bad,

but the ones that I had before that I threw up. I got real, real cold.

Dr: How often do you get these headaches?

Pt: I had two real bad ones within two weeks' time, then I didn't have none for a few weeks. Now the ones that I had last week, I didn't throw up with them, but they were enough that I had to go to bed with them.

Dr: Are the headaches something that occur almost every week, almost every month, or every couple of months?

Pt: I get them all the time. It is just within the last few months that I have been getting them more frequently. But I have averaged maybe one or two a month.

Dr: When you get these headaches, where does it hurt?

Pt: They start here and they just go around. Sometimes they'll go on one side of my face, sometimes on the other side of my face. But they start in the back of my neck here.

Dr: Do you get any kind of problems with your eyes when these headaches are coming on?

Pt: Blurred vision. The light bothers me.

Dr: Both eyes or one eye?

Pt: I have to go—like I go upstairs in my bedroom and like close everything up and I just lay down with a blanket.

Dr: What kind of problem does the light give you when you have a headache?

Pt: It just bothers me, just the light in itself, it's like a glare. The light itself bothers me.

Dr: What do these headaches keep you from doing?

Pt: Everything. I can't do a thing. When I get one, I have to go to bed. That's exactly what I do. Usually I throw up with them. I get real, real cold. It can be 90 outside, I'm freezing. Mostly the throwing up is a light vomiting.

Dr: Is there anything you can think of that triggers these headaches?

Pt: Nothing, it just starts.

Dr: Okay. What kind of person are you? Do you get pretty anxious?

Pt: Little things will set me off. Like if my kids are fighting, that bothers me, or if I feel like I'm overly tired or something like that. Little things bother me, that's all, but I've always been a nervous person.

Dr: When you get upset or you get nervous is that likely to start up your headaches? Is there any kind of connection between the two?

Pt: I can get up with a headache. If I get up with it, I'm done for the whole day. I do nothing all day.

Dr: Do these headaches scare you?

> Pt: No, I'm used to them.
> Dr: Okay, so they don't frighten you; it's just a matter of trying to . . .
> Pt: To get rid of them.

There is no unambiguous test for the etiology of headache; only a careful and precise history will distinguish between migraine and muscle contraction headaches. This physician does not accept the patient's or previous doctor's diagnosis of "migraine" headache ("What do you mean by 'migraine headaches?' ") and goes on to get many details about frequency, location, visual symptoms, and other associated symptoms.

SENSITIVITY AND SPECIFICITY

Accuracy and precision are two criteria by which we judge medical tests. Two others are sensitivity and specificity. The **sensitivity** of a test expresses its ability to "pick up" real cases of the disease in question. The higher the sensitivity, the greater the number of cases actually have a positive test result. **Specificity**, on the other hand, refers to a test's ability to "rule out" disease in normal people. The higher the specificity, the more likely a negative test result actually identifies people who do not have the disease. Few, if any, tests in medicine approach 100 percent sensitivity and specificity; certainly, your medical interview will not yield such definitive information.

A symptom may well be very sensitive (cough, in cases of pneumonia) but not specific at all (dozens of diseases cause cough); or it may be relatively specific (nocturnal mid-epigastric pain relieved by eating, in cases of duodenal ulcer) but not very sensitive (most persons with duodenal ulcer do not have that symptom). This relative lack of sensitivity and specificity for individual symptoms is one reason why physicians often minimize the value of their history taking and rush into "more scientific" tests. However, an individual symptom is not the appropriate unit on which to base decisions; we deal, rather, in symptom complexes, patterns, or pictures. We consider a detailed reconstruction of the illness, rather than isolated statements about symptoms.

A complete symptom complex may well be quite sensitive and specific, adequate, in fact, to serve as the basis for diagnosis and therapeutic decisions. Even when the "complete history" is not enough information, it is usually **most** of the information; it narrows the range of possible problems dramatically and yields a very small number of hypotheses to be supported, ruled out, or confirmed by physical examination and further studies. The well-conducted patient interview will yield a firm (and large) data base on which to design an efficient (and small) diagnostic plan. In order to achieve this result, however, the physician must approach the task objectively and precisely: the **real** sensitivity and specificity of a symptom complex are irrelevant in a given situation if the instrument through which the data are obtained (the clinician) lacks accuracy and precision.

REPRODUCIBILITY

Reproducibility is another important characteristic of "scientific" tests, including good medical interviewing. However, reproducibility of the medical history is a goal that must be tempered by several considerations about both human nature and the interactive process. In caring for a patient in the hospital, three or four observers will often obtain three or four different "versions" of that patient's history. Much of the time the differences may not be of great significance, but sometimes they will be crucial. Only one of the four observers, for example, may note that the patient has had bright-red rectal bleeding intermittently for the last three months. This fact might be lost in the review of systems and only elicited by a direct question, because the patient actually came into the hospital for chest pain and was too embarrassed to mention the bleeding spontaneously. It suddenly becomes an important issue when you find the patient has a stool positive for occult blood or a hematocrit of 32 percent. The whole team might have to shift gears from "ischemic heart disease work-up" to "lower GI bleeding work-up." Of course, just as in the laboratory, data that change from one "experiment" to the next are always suspect. Reproducibility is a characteristic highly valued in testing; its apparent lack makes many physicians question the value of medical history taking. Of course, one problem is that different history taking instruments (physicians) manifest different levels of accuracy and precision.

There are, however, several other reasons why various observers may get varying stories at different times. **First,** patients come to the hospital or to the doctor with a series of symptoms but often with no index of which symptoms are more important or less important in explaining the type or severity of their underlying disease. A severe headache may cause the patient more pain than a sudden swelling of the left leg; but the latter could be secondary to lymphatic obstruction by metastatic cancer, while the former may have no pathologic significance at all. Each time a patient is interviewed and presents a history, he or she learns what is of most importance to the interviewers. The patient will, in a sense, learn to "package" the history and make it more efficient or medically relevant or interesting to the clinician. Therefore, it is likely that later observers will get a more clearly connected and flowing—or at least different—history than the first interviewer.

Second, a corollary to this "educational" process is that patients may learn to consider some things important that they had not bothered mentioning originally. The person may have forgotten the first episode of syncope or may have considered an illness occurring three years ago as something entirely unrelated to the present one. Repetition and focusing on symptoms will not only make the story more coherent but also will refresh the patient's memory or, perhaps, set the stage for some new insight. Therefore, it is likely that later observers may pick up entirely new information that the patient neglected to mention earlier.

Third, sick people have already "organized" their illness in some way that makes sense to them, before they see the doctor (Balint, 1972). They will have tried getting rid of the symptoms on their own and perhaps will have asked for advice from family or friends. In this process, patients develop some hypothesis about what the problem is, based on personal experience or other sources of information. Consequently, patients are likely to tell their tales in ways consistent with their hypothesis; they will emphasize the symptoms that support their theory and minimize or forget those symptoms that do not. In other words, the primary data are filtered through patients' own hypotheses and beliefs. In the course of being interviewed by different people trying to direct the flow of data toward medical hypotheses, a patient's hypothesis may change. And when the primary data are filtered through a different set of beliefs, the primary data may also appear to change; the ignored or forgotten symptom may now appear.

A **fourth** reason that different histories are obtained at different times is that the patient simply and consciously "changed his story." Medical students or doctors usually invoke this reason when they dislike the patient or are unable to account for the symptoms. The more the symptoms seem to be unrelated to "objective" findings on diagnostic tests, the more likely they are to be considered imaginary and susceptible to change from one history-taking session to another. Although some patients, of course, do change their story, the so-called unreliable patient is actually a much less frequent explanation for "changing" symptoms than are the other factors we are considering.

Finally, it is clear that interviewing skills play a part as well: a physician who is empathic and asks open-ended questions is much more likely to obtain an accurate picture than a physician who asks a list of questions by rote. Skill in interviewing may bear some general relationship to the person's experience level (medical student, intern, resident, attending physician), but when one considers an individual interview of an individual patient all bets are off. The inexperienced medical student who can spend time with a patient in a nonthreatening atmosphere may learn a lot more than a hurried attending physician. In general, interviewing skills that maximize objectivity and precision reduce the rate of "false-positive" and "false-negative" histories.

THE SCIENCE AND ART OF HISTORY TAKING

As one develops clinical skill, one learns techniques to achieve objectivity and precision in gathering primary data from patients. This is good science and, what is more, it allows the patient to tell his or her story without fear of being prejudged. Objectivity demands removing your own beliefs and those of the patient to get at the primary data; it involves suspending critical judgment and accepting the patient's story as his or her unique experience. Objectivity and precision involve "understanding" or "knowing" as though it were you having the same symptom that the patient is describing. It is interesting to note that Carl Rogers defined empathy as "understanding exactly." If this is how we mean objectivity and precision, then the skills required to be objective and precise are the same skills as those required for being a nonjudgmental, compassionate, and empathic observer.

Thus, a **scientific** approach to history taking permits and reinforces an **artful** approach to the patient. Is there not a contradiction between a "just get the facts" history and an empathic history? We would argue that there is no such contradiction, that you cannot "get the facts" without understanding and without suspending judgment. If you do, the "facts" that you get may not be the relevant facts. You will begin a vicious cycle in which, since your history provides such poor information, you will undervalue history taking and rely more and more on a "shotgun" approach to diagnostic tests. A good scientific history is at the same time an empathic or "artful" one. The two result from facets of the same skill, as shown in Figure 1. To get the facts, you must understand and not judge; if you do otherwise you will lose primary data essential to making the diagnosis. And when you understand and are nonjudgmental, your interview will build rapport—often the start of a therapeutic relationship—and will gather the data that tells not only **what** the diagnosis is but also **who** the patient is.

A patient says this best. The following is part of an interview in which the patient describes how it feels to be understood and not judged:

Pt: Aw, I'm not usually this able to talk to people like this. I don't really know you . . .

Dr: That's true. I'm a total stranger.

Pt: And all of a sudden I have gone completely down the line and told you everything I could possibly think of to tell you. I've never been able to do that, I have very few people that I talk to personally or talk to about the way I feel . . . um . . . I talk to my family but there are only certain things that you can talk to your family about, and I have never had anyone I could talk to, I have always kept everything to myself. And now, all of a sudden, I've just flowed over like a broken toilet.

Dr: Was it helpful?

Pt: Yes, because I just learned something else about myself. The

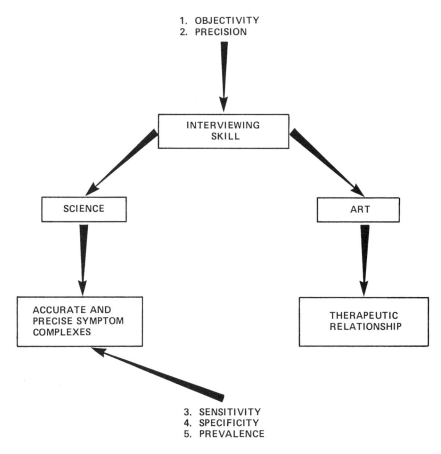

FIGURE 1. General components of medical interviewing.

funny thing is, I have said all these things to you and most times talking to people, I always think before I talk. I have said everything I have said to you without thinking about it first, and without wondering what you are going to think about what I am saying to you. And I can honestly say that I have never done that with anyone.

Dr: Uh huh.

Pt: I . . . um . . . have, maybe, I have a lot of friends but I mean, people you can really sit down and tell every little thing that happens in your life. There are very very few of those. And I even, I even think before I say what I say to them because there's always a chance that someone misinterprets and, really deep down I always know I want their opinion because I know they

> are my friends, and they are going to say what I want to hear
> and that's not always what I need to hear.
> Dr: Well, I'm glad. Because I like to think it's helpful.
> Pt: It really is. I feel quite good about the whole thing.

The patient here describes being able to say everything "without thinking about it first." What he is describing is his ability to reveal uncensored primary data that are vital to the diagnostic process; what permitted him to do this was not "wondering what you are going to think about what I am saying to you." This is the aim of medical interviewing and history taking. Revealing uncensored data was crucial for this patient, who presented with a rash that proved to be secondary syphilis acquired in the course of multiple homosexual contacts. Had the patient filtered out data about his sexual activity, the diagnosis would have been made less quickly or, perhaps, not at all.

In this book, you will learn to improve the equipment with which you examine patients, namely yourselves. You will learn how to listen and how to use words. We will not describe symptom complexes in detail, estimate their sensitivity and specificity, or list the prevalence of various diseases; one learns these from courses on pathophysiology and medicine and from the experience of seeing many patients. Likewise, we will not focus much on the **structure** of history taking, at least in the sense of "which questions to ask for which disease." The traditional outline of a medical history is rather rigidly defined—chief complaint, present illness, past medical history, family history, social history, review of systems; lists of questions and hypotheses to consider, as in Kraytman's *The Complete Medical History* (1979), describe the possible content and structure of a medical history. The traditional outline presents one way of recording data you obtain, and it is useful to review after the interview to see if there are pertinent questions that you did not ask. However, the traditional outline is not the "how" of getting the information. It is the "how" that concerns us here. You will learn how to ask questions so that patients understand what you mean; for example, you would not ask most patients (unless they are medical students), "Do you have dysuria?" but rather "Does it hurt to pass your water?" You will learn **how** to gain the patient's continued cooperation in obtaining data, how to organize complex information, and how to guide confusing stories. And you will observe the effect of the doctor-patient interaction on the quality of the historic data as well as on the management of the patient and his or her illness.

SAGA OF THE FIFTH WHEEL

This section is an aside to address certain concerns of students who are just beginning to learn patient interviewing and physical examination. Often in a hospital setting, where the patients are quite ill, the beginning student feels like a sort of spare part, a "fifth wheel," someone who has no responsibility for patients' care. Besides simple inexperience and the anxiety associated with it, this situation leads students to have several other realistic concerns about interacting with patients to whom they are assigned. Three of the major ones are: (1) I don't know enough about pathophysiology to do a good history and physical examination, let alone to "get" the diagnosis; (2) the patients have been worked over 10 times already and are generally tired of it all, and sometimes angry, by the time I come in to examine them; and (3) I have no responsibility for the patient, nor the ability to help, so I feel like an interloper—a "fifth wheel."

Of course, each of these has an element of truth, but none of them need be a major constraint in your interviewing and physical diagnosis experience. Let us deal with each concern.

First, "I don't know enough pathophysiology." It is clear that you are not going to characterize patterns of symptoms as well or as efficiently as an experienced physician; nor will you be able to "pick up" the subtle physical signs. You might, for example, examine a patient with peptic ulcer before you have studied the gastrointestinal tract in your pathophysiology course. You will complain: "I don't know what symptoms to ask about. I don't know what direction to take." As long as the final **content** of the history (or physical) is all that interests you, there is no way to get beyond your lack of knowledge. However, the clinical art (and the point of this book) is to learn the **process** and **method.** Your goal is to learn to talk with patients in a way in which you can maximize both information gathering and therapeutic communication (Fig. 1). The diagnosis (although interesting) is largely irrelevant at this point—you are not expected to make good diagnostic hypotheses without a knowledge of relevant pathophysiology. Your goal is to characterize the symptoms and the person as precisely and objectively as possible and, more importantly, to create an interview situation in which this can occur.

Wolraich and co-workers conducted a study to determine whether improvement in knowledge about medical conditions or disease processes improves the students' interviewing skills (Wolraich et al, 1982). They assigned 10 students to an experimental group that received some intensive education about diagnosis and management of meningomyelocele; a control group of 10 students did not receive this information. Each subject in both groups then interviewed in a simulated clinical situation the mother of a child with meningomyelocele, and each interaction was rated for interviewing skills and informational content. They found that the students' interviewing skills were not affected by an increase in their knowledge about the medical condition. Other studies have suggested, in fact, that the interviewing skills of medical students tend to decline as they progress from their first to their fourth year of medical education (Wright et al,

1980). This is certainly consistent with our experience as preceptors and attending physicians. We give these examples only to point out that, at the very least, the question of whether specific medical knowledge improves the process of interviewing is an unresolved one.

Second, "the patients have often had numerous other examinations and are sick and tired of it all." The anger your patient expresses (or just barely conceals) very frequently arises not from the mere fact of repeated examinations, but from the whole situation—being ill, having a backache that no one pays attention to, uncomfortable diagnostic studies, doctors who are rude or preoccupied, nurses who seem unsympathetic, and so forth. The anger is there even before you arrive on the scene.

How do you deal with this? It is crucial to clarify your role, not just as a student, but as a student learning to do an interview, someone who will *not* be taking care of the patient on the hospital unit. Then, make sure the patient has really consented to your interview and examination. If he or she does not wish to talk with you and says so, let it go at that. For patients who are tired or in pain, suggest the possibility of your coming in later; if the patient seems angry, acknowledge the anger. This will give you a good opportunity to see how effective "interchangeable" responses can be (see Chapter 2, section on "Levels of Responding") in obtaining information and developing rapport.

Sick people, like anyone else, may have several mutually conflicting feelings at the same time. A given patient may want to be helpful to a student, angry about the situation, depressed about being ill, and simply all tired out—simultaneously. You can tip the balance in your favor: by being straight with the patient and really listening, you will avoid contributing to the patient's anger and will also tend to defuse it.

Third, "I can't help this patient." The whole issue of responsibility and helpfulness needs another look. The professional role is not something you put on overnight when you get your degree. You grow into it. As a medical student you are demonstrably more a physician now than you were two years ago; as a nursing student you are clearly more a nurse now than you were two years ago. Although a learner, you are interacting with patients in a professional manner. The information you gather is important. Although the disease data you collect only occasionally contributes to what physicians have already gathered, the person data you collect will often contribute. If the patient has a specific request or complaint, you can discuss it with a unit nurse or with the medical resident. If the patient has a misunderstanding, you can clarify it or find somebody else to do so.

Finally, simply listening to patients in an empathic manner is therapeutic. It might not repair the damaged myocardium or lower the blood sugar, but it will make the patient feel better. That is, after all, what medicine is all about, although the goal of helping another human being to feel better often becomes confused (or at least remote) in a modern hospital. The patient is in a strange environment with a potentially serious or life-threatening illness and is caught in a system (the hospital) that is not always flexible or responsive to the patient's needs. If you are willing to take the time to listen, you will be surprised how therapeutic the encounter with you is for your patient, even though you are ostensibly "doing nothing."

CHAPTER 2

Fundamental Skills: Understanding Exactly

A very good way to find out what another person is thinking or feeling is to ask him . . . At this point, however, a difficulty arises. If I am to acquire information in this way about another person's experiences, I must understand what he says about them. And this would seem to imply that I attach the same meaning to his words as he does. But how, it may be asked, can I ever be sure that this is so?

Alfred Jules Ayer, *The Problem of Knowledge*

Almost everyone agrees that certain attitudes toward patients are praiseworthy; they include such qualities as genuineness and empathy. On first hearing, these sound like basic attitudes reflecting the doctor's personality and value structure. They do not sound like concepts immediately relevant to taking a medical history, particularly not "skills" that can be learned and manipulated in dealing with patients. However, these qualities can be defined and observed as a certain set of behaviors. These behaviors can be taught, practiced, and learned.

In this chapter we borrow some concepts from psychologists, particularly Carl Rogers and his followers, who first identified certain observable qualities of the therapist or helper, qualities that correlated with good therapeutic outcomes. They called these **therapeutic core qualities,** and the three most important were **respect** (or unconditional positive regard), **genuineness** (or congruence), and **empathy.** They found that the content of psychotherapeutic intervention, such as the specific interventions dictated by a theory, was less important to success than the process of the interactions. Subsequently, other investigators defined specific skills evident in that process. They showed that qualities such as empathy could be broken down into a set of skills in listening to and responding to a patient (Ivey and Authier, 1978).

These "therapeutic core qualities" are important links between the art and science of medicine. They are pertinent to this text, because they improve history-taking ability and the accuracy of the data obtained, and because they lead to better therapeutic relationships in ordinary practice. In the last chapter, we identified the goal of maximizing objectivity and precision in our communication with patients. In this chapter, we will look at some "generic" concepts about how to do this, before taking up the actual skills of medical history taking. The following two examples serve to introduce these concepts. One is of a practicing physician interviewing a new patient in his office; the other is of a medical intern taking the history of his new patient in the clinic. In the first example, the patient is a 50-year-old woman who complains chiefly of abdominal pain that is worse when she is "upset":

Dr: What happens when you get upset? What do you feel like?

Pt: Oh, I just feel **right nervous**, the stomach pains, my arm . . . it pains, it seems like the strength is going out of my arm and hands.

Dr: How often do you get upset?

Pt: Quite frequently.

Dr: What's quite frequent?

Pt: Mostly every day it seems like I'm upset. **I get something on my mind** and that brings on the nauseated feeling.

Dr: So what's the usual sequence? You get upset first and then what happens? You get upset first or does the nausea come on first?

Pt: No. I get upset and then the nausea comes on.

Dr: What are you upset about?

Pt: Well, you know, things you want around the house there . . . it seems like things don't go right around the house. Like I get upset about that.

Dr: Tell me about when you started being upset.

Pt: Oh really, right after my mother passed, really, in April, I've been mostly upset.

Dr: What happened when your mother passed away? I understand it must have been a very upsetting event; was she very close to you?

Pt: Yes, I was really close to my mother, and it seems like after she passed, I don't know, something just left out of me, I don't know what it was, you know.

In the second example, the patient is a 40-year-old man who came for a "check-up." The doctor is inquiring about his family history and found that the patient's father had died of a ruptured aneurysm in the brain.

Dr: You don't know anything more about that?

Pt: Well, my understanding is, the context of this is, that my mother was raised in the Catholic Church, and divorce was a terrible scandal in her mind and she tried to forget about it as quickly as she could. It's such a painful subject that there was never any discussion about who he was and so forth. And as a consequence all I've really heard are niblets, and one of the things I understand is that my father was an alcoholic or at least he had a problem with alcohol, but really caused my mother a lot of problems. So, I don't know if that could be a complicating factor in terms of an aneurysm or not.

Dr: Not that I know of. How about brothers and sisters?

Pt: I have one full natural brother and then four half brothers.

Dr: Medical problems in any of them that you know of?

Pt: No.

Dr: And you work as?

Pt: An editorial writer for the *Journal*.

Dr: And coming through your summer jobs, any unusual exposure to chemicals or mills or anything unusual that you did?

Pt: No, I worked in a bakery.

Dr: Asbestos?

All we have are transcripts of the tape-recorded histories, so we cannot reconstruct the tone or quality of language, or the nonverbal communication. However, the doctor in the first example (who, by the way, is the medical intern) appears to be "connecting" with his patient. He acknowledges both the facts that he is getting and also the feelings ("I understand it must have been a very upsetting event"). The doctor in our second example does not appear to be on the same wavelength with his patient. He is following his own agenda with little regard for the other person. The patient has told the doctor that his father died of a cerebral hemorrhage but does not know anything else about it because his parents were divorced. The divorce, the "painful subject," and the history of alcoholism that pours out are ignored by the doctor who abruptly answers the patient's overt question and moves on ("Not that I know of. How about brothers and sisters?"). The second excerpt gives us a feeling that (at least in this interview) the doctor's history taking—in particular, his ability to do it with empathy and respect—leaves something to be desired.

We define three important skills that enhance communication between doctor and patient as follows:

RESPECT. The ability to accept the patient as a unique person, suspending critical judgment; accepting the patient as he or she is.

GENUINENESS. The ability to be oneself in a relationship, not hiding behind a role or façade.

EMPATHY. The ability to sense the patient's experience and feelings accurately, as well as to communicate that understanding back to the patient.

Respect, genuineness, and empathy are qualities that we demonstrate in relationships with our patients by using certain techniques of communication. An important skill in dealing with patients is to maximize your ability to display these qualities through your behavior on any given occasion. When patients feel understood and respected, we greatly increase our chances of obtaining accurate primary data. We look next at each skill and discuss specific ways to communicate to patients that we understand and respect them.

RESPECT

Respect means to value individuals' traits and beliefs despite one's own personal feelings about them, to see patients' habits or feelings as their best adaptation to their illness or life circumstances. Clearly, this is a crucial issue in medicine. Some patients have habits such as smoking cigarettes, drinking too much, refusing to take medications and even, at times, being antagonistic to their doctors or to medical students. Other patients have beliefs about their illnesses that try our patience: the patient with severe emphysema may explain to you that his illness has nothing to do with his 100 pack-year smoking history but was caused by a cold he never got rid of in 1956. Another patient might drive you up the wall with devastating migratory pains that never go away. Some patients may be unable to keep themselves clean or will be grossly obese. Many will have different value systems from yours or a healthy skepticism about medical technology.

The skill in having respect is to separate your personal feelings about the patient's behavior or attitudes or beliefs from your fundamental concern about helping him or her get well. For example, the patient who believes that his emphysema is unrelated to smoking can still be guided to give a reliable account of his own symptoms. Likewise, while the hostile patient will make you feel uncomfortable, you can still try to respect her reasons for being angry. Moreover, the emphysema patient's denial and the hostile patient's anger may actually be vital to their ability to tolerate being ill; such feelings must be accepted as part of the whole patient, not rejected as threats to the ego of the physician.

Respect involves those skills that demonstrate valuing the patient as a person and as a historian. The following case example, taken from Platt and McMath (1979) demonstrates lack of respect in several ways.

The interviewer failed to knock at the patient's door. He introduced himself in a hasty mumble so that the patient never had his name clearly in mind. He mispronounced the patient's name once and never used it again. The physician conducted the interview while seated in a chair about 7 feet from the patient. There was no physical contact during the interview. On several occasions the patient expressed her emotional distress. On each occasion the interviewer ignored the emotional content of her statements.

Dr: Exactly where is this pain?
Pt: It's so hard for me to explain. I'm trying to do as well as I can. *(Turning to husband)* Aren't I doing as well as I can?
Dr: Well, is the pain up high in your belly, or down low?
Pt: I kept getting weaker and weaker. I didn't want to come to the hospital. I was so frightened *(weeping)*.
Dr: Did the pain come before the weakness or afterward?

The physical examination was brusque, the examiner never warning his patient when painful maneuvers (for example, stroking the sole of the foot) were to be done. At the end of the examination the physician failed to comment on his findings or his plans. He said in parting, "We'll do some tests and see if we can find out just what's the matter with you," and left the room before the patient had an opportunity to question him.

Notice how the physician seems to have his own agenda, ignoring the patient both as a person (by not acknowledging her emotional distress) and as a historian (by not helping to clarify the nature of the pain and weakness). This vignette illustrates a number of simple things you can do to demonstrate respect for your patient. **First,** you can introduce yourself clearly and communicate specifically why you are there. Since you are not the patient's friend, it would demonstrate lack of respect to use his or her first name during an initial interview. **Second,** you could inquire about and arrange for the patient's comfort before getting started, and continue to consider his or her comfort during the course of your history and physical examination. **Third,** you can conduct the interview while sitting at the patient's level in a position where you can be easily seen and heard. **Fourth,** you can warn the patient when you intend to do or say something unexpected or painful, particularly in the physical examination. **Finally,** you can respond to your patient in a way that indicates you have heard what he or she has said. The previous interview might have gone something like this:

Dr: Exactly where is this pain?
Pt: It's so hard for me to explain. I'm trying to do as well as I can.

> *(Turning to husband)* Aren't I doing as well as I can?
>
> Dr: I can see it's hard for you to explain and that you're trying hard. Perhaps you can show me where you are feeling it right now.
>
> Pt: It's right about here but what really frightened me was that I kept getting weaker and weaker and I didn't want to come to the hospital *(weeping)*.
>
> Dr: *(Handing patient a box of tissues)* Here, do you need one of these? Was it the weakness that frightened you?

Now the physician is focusing not only on the symptoms but also on the patient's feelings about the symptoms. In so doing, he is likely to communicate his respect for the patient; he is also more likely to acquire accurate data and to do so more efficiently.

GENUINENESS

Genuineness means not pretending to be somebody or something other than who or what you are; it means being yourself, both as the person who you are and as the professional that you are. The first time you encounter this concept of genuineness as a problem in medicine may be with regard to your role as a physical diagnosis or medical interviewing student. How do you introduce yourself? Should you introduce yourself as a medical student or as a doctor? Do you allow a patient to address you as doctor? How do you respond when patients ask you medical questions beyond your expertise, or inquire about their own prognosis or care? Or when they say, "You look too young to be a doctor!" In all these cases if you are to be genuine, you must acknowledge what you are: a **medical student.** You should introduce yourself as a medical student and, wherever appropriate, reaffirm to the patient your limited medical knowledge and limited responsibility (but not limited interest!) in the patient's case. This does not mean you should avoid being helpful by, for example, transmitting the patient's requests to the unit physicians, obtaining medical information for the patient from his or her doctor, or encouraging the patient to ask the question you are unable to answer of someone who can help.

The term **student doctor** may represent a useful concept, both for you and for the patient. It acknowledges the patient's need—as well as your own—to perceive you in a professional, helping role, while it also genuinely describes what you are. "Student doctor" more closely defines your role when you are talking with patients than does the more nondescript term "medical student." It also allows you to experience yourself in a more professional light and may facilitate your helping attitude toward the patient.

Interns, residents, and physicians in practice all experience situations in which their patients ask for opinions or require procedures beyond their capabilities. They are required to call in consultants or refer their patients to specialists. This does not mean abandoning patients when their problems exceed your area of expertise. In such instances, being genuine means outlining what you do and do not know, or can and cannot do, and negotiating a plan for future care that involves, for example, consulting a specialist.

Being genuine also means being yourself in another way, that of expressing your feelings while staying within the bounds of a professional relationship. If a patient is in the hospital for a medical or surgical illness but has experienced a recent loss, such as the death of a spouse, it is not only reasonable but even desirable to respond to this fact with a statement such as, "I am sorry to hear that. How has it been going for you?" However, adding that you too have lost a spouse may stress the limits of what you feel comfortable with in a professional relationship. When patients say or describe things that are sad or funny it is appropriate to respond as a person and not just as a history-taking machine. Demonstrating your interest in the patient as a person is another way of being genuine.

Everyone has bad days, and you may happen to be at a low ebb yourself during your evaluation of the patient. You may have been on call and up all night with a patient in the intensive care unit. You may be having problems in your personal life or eagerly anticipating a weekend of skiing when you leave the hospital. At other times, you may be outraged about the patient's behavior, such as her canceling or coming late to appointments. What is the role of "genuineness" in these situations? Should you hide your feelings, disguise your bad day, or express them to the patient? Genuineness means not pretending, but it does **not** mean that you must share all your feelings with the patient. You must distinguish your genuine **professional self** from the vicissitudes, experiences, or interests of your **personal self.** As you go through medical school and residency, you gradually develop your professional self into a well-integrated instrument of healing. It is this professional self that serves as the standard for your genuineness. For example, the patient who makes you angry by continually canceling or coming late to appointments can be told that you (as a person) are angry about that, but (as a professional) you try to confine your anger to that aspect of the relationship. At the same time, you try to respect the patient by understanding the patient's reasons for being late (chaotic lifestyle, three children under the age of 5, single parenting, need to take three buses to get there, and so forth). This does not mean that you are not being genuine; rather, you are being your professional, helping self. Understanding is a prerequisite to respecting; the more you understand the more likely that your respect will be genuine.

This leads to two caveats. **First,** it is rarely helpful to share your personal anger or disgust with the patient in the name of being honest. You may confront the patient with inconsistencies (to you) in his story, or point out his erratic behavior, if you believe it will help therapeutically; this is not the same as sharing your own negative feelings. **Second,** sometimes physicians are tempted to share their experiences and feelings as illustrations for the patient. This may range from statements like "I have young children too, and I know what you mean," to detailed personal anecdotes. Here again it is crucial to judge your personal revelations in the light of your professional judgment. Ordinarily, comments of rapport and "connection" are helpful. The type of car you own, the vagaries of parenting, or your opinions about a football team are not really self-revelations. On the other hand, it is rarely part of a genuine doctor-patient interaction to describe intimate experiences or specific political or moral values.

EMPATHY AND LEVELS OF RESPONDING

Empathy

Empathy is understanding; it is not an emotional state of feeling sympathy or feeling sorry for someone. In taking a medical history, being empathic means listening to the total communication—words, feelings, gestures—and letting the patient know that you are hearing what he or she is saying. The empathic physician is also the scientific physician, because understanding is also the core concept of objectivity. The empathic scientific physician is the one most likely to obtain an accurate history.

There are certain ways of responding to what patients say that will help you demonstrate that you understand. The skill in being objective/ empathic is in learning how to talk to patients to maximize your ability to gather accurate data. The data about life circumstances and specific symptoms that the patient gives you will be associated with feelings and beliefs. Remember the maxim, "you don't speak to patients; you speak to a set of beliefs about the world" (Cassell, 1979). The patient who gives you a detailed description of her abdominal pain may at the same time feel frightened because she fears the pain means stomach cancer since her father died of stomach cancer. Her description will be filtered through her fear and her belief; unless you attend to the worry, the patient may not give an accurate account of what she is actually experiencing. One patient may magnify the symptom to ensure a complete work-up that will not miss cancer; another may minimize the symptom in hope of being reassured. If the interviewer acknowledges the fear, it is easier to find out what is really going on and get accurate data.

An empathic response can also be important in helping the patient to clarify what he or she is feeling. At times the patient will not be in touch with his or her own feelings. By checking within yourself—"How would I feel in this situation (for instance, finding blood in my stool)?"—you can formulate a response. Then by checking back with the patient—"That can be pretty frightening"—you as the interviewer can find out whether your assessment of what the patient might have felt is valid in that person's experience of illness. The patient might agree that he or she was frightened or might say, as in the case of someone with chronic ulcerative colitis, "No, I didn't feel frightened, because I knew what it was, but I was frustrated (or angry) because everything was going along well and I really thought I'd licked the problem." Even if the patient disagrees with your initial formulation of the feeling response, you have opened the way for the patient to talk freely about his or her feelings. At the same time you have gathered additional data about this person's experience of illness.

Levels of Responding

If the patient believes that you are picking up on everything he or she says and are listening attentively with a nonjudgmental attitude, not only will accurate data emerge but feelings and beliefs as well. In formulating a response it is important first to assess the nature and intensity of any feeling expressed; for example, is the patient upset? And if upset, is he or she slightly upset or furious? Your assessment will include not only what the patient says but how it is said and how the patient looks at the time. Your assessment of the strength of the feeling that the patient is experiencing will influence what you say to the patient.

To talk to patients you have to learn a professional way of responding, different from the way you might respond in social interactions. In social situations we often ignore or minimize feelings; for example, when people say "How are you?" or "How do you feel today?" they do not ordinarily expect you to reveal how lousy you are actually feeling. In the clinical setting, however, you really do want to know how the person is feeling; you acknowledge the intensity of any feelings expressed and demonstrate that you understand and accept these feelings.

One way to assess how to respond is to consider certain categories or "levels" of responding:

1. **Ignoring.** You either do not hear what the patient has said or act as though you did not hear. There is no response to either the symptom content or feelings.
   Examples:
   (a) Pt: Most days my arthritis is so bad the swelling and pain are just too much.
       Dr: And have you ever had any operations?
   (b) Dr: Do things emotional at work seem to make it worse?
       Pt: I think it's . . .

> Dr: Do coughing, sneezing, bending, straining at stool, any of those things make it worse?
> Pt: I never associated it with those things.

2. **Minimizing.** You respond to the feelings and symptoms at less than the actual level expressed by the patient.
   Examples:
   (a) Pt: I was in agony with the pain and terribly frightened.
   >   Dr: So you had a little pain and anxiety.
   (b) Dr: Do you feel it's getting worse or staying about the same?
   >   Pt: It's staying about the same.
   >   Dr: What are you doing for it now?
   >   Pt: Nothing. I could have went back to my doctor, you know, but he doesn't take the medical card so that's why I made an appointment to come here.
   >   Dr: Fine, I understand. How about your right leg? How has that been feeling?

3. **Interchangeable.** You recognize the feelings and symptoms expressed by the patient and assess them accurately, and you feed back that awareness at the same level of intensity.
   Example:
   > Pt: Most days my arthritis is so bad the swelling and pain are just too much. I can't seem to do anything at all any more and nothing seems to help.
   > Dr: It sounds as though the pain and disability are really getting to you.

The basic goal in medical history taking is that of the interchangeable response. This is usually a restatement in your own words of what the patient is trying to describe in order to communicate to the patient that you understand. When you give an interchangeable response, you are likely to find that this has a positive effect on the patient's ability to give an accurate history and to talk about what he or she is feeling. This kind of response is essential to being empathic. In the following dialogue, the doctor responds to her patient's concerns even though she does not answer all the patient's questions right away:

> Pt: But other than that I'm pretty good but my breasts I'm worried about. They started bleeding again, doctor, why? I want you to take a look today. They're all bleeding in the inside. Is it anything to be concerned about?
> Dr: Well maybe I can look and tell you.
> Pt: Okay.

Dr: When did that start up again?

Pt: It seems like it will come and it will go but now they're both all red and I noticed a whole lot of blood just drained out especially this right one, it really hurts down in here. This side don't hurt me but this side hurts me. I don't know.

Dr: So you want me to take a look at your breasts. *(Interchangeable response)* Is that what's worrying you most today, your breasts? Is there anything else?

Pt: No.

Dr: Okay, come and let me take a look. *(Patient and doctor move to examination table, and she begins checking patient.)* Okay, I can see why you're so concerned, it looks pretty raw here. Okay, this is pretty much like it was before.

Pt: Yeah, but it really does hurt.

Dr: Yeah, I can see that it hurts. *(Interchangeable response)* This one is the worst, huh? Remember how well we were able to clear it up with medication the last time it got this bad.

Pt: Wonder what causes that? That's what worries me.

Dr: Yes, most women do worry about things that happen to their breasts. *(Interchangeable response)* But this is not serious, although it's very annoying and painful. It's more like a skin allergy. The skin is real sensitive.

Pt: Oh, is that what it is?

There is a fourth level of responding called **additive**, in which you recognize not only what the patient expresses openly but also what he or she may be feeling and is unable to express. One common activity of physicians that involves using additive responses is that of reassurance (see Chapter 10). This involves making an educated guess regarding what the patient is likely to be worried about and dealing specifically with those worries. Here is an example of an additive response:

Dr: Well, how are you? Better? Are you having headaches?

Pt: Saturday I had a bad one. I wasn't able to sleep for five nights; my system is so pumped up I can't sleep. The sleeping pills did work. I took one a couple of hours before I went to bed and one when just, when I went to bed.

Dr: Is it the Dalmane, the kind I gave you before you went to the hospital? Is it a red and yellow capsule?

Pt: Yeah. I took them two nights and last night was the first night I could sleep without them. I don't like to take a lotta stuff. I was having very strange effects from some of the medication.

Dr: Like what?

Pt: Well, you know everything else about me, I might as well tell you this. Those green pills made me . . . well, I can't describe the feeling it made me feel . . . very strange. They also depressed me, believe it or not, even though you told me that they were antidepressants. I got depressed with them. For two days when I was taking them straight and in heavy doses, I found myself breaking into tears in situations . . . I don't even cry when I want to *(laughs)*. It was very, very strange so I stopped taking them.

Dr: So you're off them now?

Pt: Yeah, off everything now.

Dr: Okay. Can you tell me anything more about this strange feeling you had?

Pt: Ah.

Dr: **You were feeling like you were going to lose your mind?** *(Additive response)*

Pt: Yeah, I felt like I didn't have control over myself. I started to think I would get complications from the illness and how far behind it was making me get in my work because this is a very crucial time in my business. It really opened a lot of stuff for me. I never felt like this before.

The ability to achieve an additive response comes with the experience of seeing patterns of symptoms and of feelings in many patients over time. For our patient with arthritis, an additive response might be:

Pt: Most days my arthritis is so bad the swelling and pain are just too much.

Dr: It sounds as though the pain is so bad that you think that things won't get much better.

If you have not gotten the sense of the statement quite right the patient may respond:

Pt: Well, I do feel pretty bad, but I'm still hopeful.

USING WORDS TO IDENTIFY SYMPTOMS AND FEELINGS

Symptom Words

In order to increase your skill in responding appropriately to your patients, it is necessary to pay attention to words, both your own and the patient's. Premedical education and medical school can sterilize your vocabulary. You become immersed in the language of medicine, which, although very precise in describing physical attributes, leaves little room for feelings or emotions. It is a language in which adjectives and adverbs carry little weight, and you are usually discouraged from using them in conversation. This socialization into the factual language of medicine can present real problems when you speak with patients. Most vibrant, creative human beings do not happen to be medical students, doctors, or biologic scientists. The world of the sick differs from the world of the well, but the difference does not include the sick learning the language of medicine. The most obvious problem you encounter with your medical vocabulary is that patients do not understand the words you use. You may talk about hematemesis rather than vomiting up blood, or paresthesias rather than pins-and-needles sensations in the fingers. Here is an example of a medical faculty member who was trying to ask his patient how much alcohol he drank:

> Dr: Okay. Do you use ethanol a lot, little, weekends . . . ?
> Pt: Tylenol?
> Dr: Daily?
> Pt: Ethanol? Alcohol?
> Dr: Drinks?
> Pt: You mean . . . alcoholic beverages? . . . I usually have a drink every night.
> Dr: Okay.

That doctor was thinking "use ethanol" rather than "drink alcohol," and it created some (in this case, temporary) confusion. Fortunately, the patient acknowledged the misunderstanding. Many times patients do not let on that they have not understood the physician's statement. This is a particular problem with yes/no questions and with explanations/instructions in which no response is sought from the patient.

Feeling Words, Qualifiers, and Quantifiers

Another important result of medical language and thought patterns is our often-impoverished ability to describe feelings, qualities, and emotions with any accuracy or precision. Empathy requires both accurate understanding and feeding back this understanding to the patient. This demands that we identify not only facts but also feelings, not only quantities but also qualities, not only events but also emotions. We must, in a sense, open up our doors and windows to the world; we must relearn and practice using a broad vocabulary of feeling words. Patients use words to quantify many symptoms: how much pain, how much blood, how much suffering, how much vomiting. Although we are more comfortable with numbers as quantities, the patient who describes the pain as being as severe as the pain he had with his kidney stone is giving us as precise a description as the patient who says that the pain is an 8 on a scale of 1 to 10—perhaps even

TABLE 1. Descriptive Words for Levels of Feeling

	Anger	Joy	Anxiety/Fear	Depression
WEAK	Annoyed	Pleased	Uneasy	Sad
	Upset	Glad	Uncertain	Down
	Irritated	Happy	Apprehensive	Blue
MEDIUM	Angry	Turned on	Worried	Gloomy
	Testy	Joyful	Troubled	Sorrowful
	Quarrelsome	Delighted	Afraid	Miserable
STRONG	Infuriated	Marvelous	Tormented	Distraught
	Spiteful	Jubilant	Frantic	Overwhelmed
	Enraged	Ecstatic	Terrified	Devastated

more precise, as we may not know what a "10" is for him, but we do know that renal colic is one of the most severe pains a person can have.

Table 1 presents examples of words that describe various emotions and their intensity. In giving an interchangeable response to the patient, you must "hit" not only the right feeling but also the right intensity of feeling. The patient who says "I am devastated by this pain" is not likely to believe you have really heard him if your response is, "So the pain upsets you a little?" On the other hand, when the patient mentions that "I feel a little crummy today," the doctor is not sticking to her observations if she replies, "Sounds like you're feeling utterly hopeless." Once we accept the idea that medicine is about helping people to **feel** better as well as to **function** better, it is easy to understand how feelings reveal important data about the patient, which must be described as accurately and precisely as possible. Appendix A presents a long list of adjectives and adverbs that describe feelings.

NONVERBAL COMMUNICATION

Nonverbal communication is the process of transmitting information without the use of words. It includes **the way a person uses his or her body:** facial expressions, eye contact, hand and arm gestures, posture, and various movements of the legs and feet. Nonverbal communication also includes **paralinguistics** or the "how" of speech; this encompasses voice qualities, the speed at which a person talks, silent pauses, and speech errors. It is probably through the nonverbal aspects of communication that we apprehend another's feelings. We recognize anger not so much by what a person says as by how it is said; speech may slow down and get quiet—"controlled" anger—or the opposite may occur with shouting and gestures, such as pounding the fist. We can often tell when people lie, unless they are good liars; often they will look away, break eye contact, hesitate, get "red in the face"—an involuntary flush. Common medical examples are the pressure of speech in the anxious or hypomanic person, or the dead voice tone of the very depressed. Patients who are ill often "sound" weak; we may gauge a person's state of health by how he or she sounds ("She's been through a lot of surgery, but she really sounds strong!").

Another component of nonverbal communication involves the **use of personal and social space;** how physically close do we get while talking to our friends, business associates, lovers, patients. Other factors such as personal grooming, clothing, and odors (for example, perspiration, alcohol, tobacco) also communicate information about the patient without words and can be helpful to you in your understanding of the patient. For example, if a patient who is normally careful about personal grooming and dress comes in disheveled and unkempt, you are alerted to the possibility of a problem.

Much of the patient's nonverbal communication, while obvious to you, will be concealed from the patient. This does not mean that the messages sent nonverbally are invalid; in fact, they may be more accurate than the verbal message, because the nonverbal message is often sent unintentionally and uncensored. Although it is interesting to note various aspects of nonverbal communication, you may wonder what to do with your observations. The main feature to look for is **consistency;** note nonverbal behaviors and determine whether or not they are congruent with the patient's verbal message. When there is congruence between verbal and nonverbal messages, the communication is more or less straightforward; when there is a discrepancy, an effort must be made to ascertain which is the real message.

Here is an example of a patient who came in for a routine follow-up of abdominal pain and reported first that her husband, from whom she was separated, died recently of some sudden and unknown reason (he was 27 years old). David is the child they had together.

> Pt: I want to tell you something before we start.
> Dr: Okay.
> Pt: David's dad died.
> Dr: Ah-h-h.
> Pt: And now, it's like every week it's something new.
> Dr: Oh my. What happened?
> Pt: I don't know. He just went to sleep and never woke up.
> Dr: My goodness, when did that happen?
> Pt: Last Friday, right before the 9th.
> Dr: Oh, I am so sorry to hear that. Ah, how is David doing?

The physician went on to explore how the patient and her son were reacting to this event, but all the while the patient was discussing things with a bright smile on her face. Although she was separated from her husband, they had remained close and cordial because of David, and her cheeriness seemed inappropriate. Indeed, it later came out that she was having great difficulty, particularly in communicating to her son appropriate ways to both mourn and remember his father.

Often the nonverbal message will be more accurate than the verbal statements made. In some situations, especially early in the interview, you may choose simply to note a discrepancy and use it to help you understand the patient. Or you might use the nonverbal communication to modify your own nonverbal behavior or your conversation or both. For example, if the patient seems tense and anxious, as evidenced by flushing or fidgeting, you may modify your voice tone and the way you are sitting in response to the patient's discomfort.

At the same time that you are observing the patient's nonverbal behavior, the patient is, perhaps unconsciously, observing your nonverbal behavior as well. As a result, your job is twofold; you should be aware of the patient's nonverbal behaviors as well as your own. For example, if you seem uninterested, as evidenced by never looking at the patient or by looking at your watch, the patient may be unable to provide the details you need. Attention to your own nonverbal behavior requires a high level of self-awareness as you conduct the interview. It is particularly important to be conscious of how you respond to distractions during the interview, such as an emergency going on across the hall. You need to demonstrate your focus on the patient by maintaining eye contact, an attentive posture, and a seeming lack of awareness that all hell is breaking loose somewhere else.

Gestures

Although many specific **gestures** have been subject to study and suggested interpretations, these must always be judged in the context of the entire situation and confirmed with the patient. When the gesture or facial expression appears to imply something different than the words, an effort must be made to ascertain which—gesture or words—is delivering the real message. The nonverbal message may be more accurate. Interpretation is no problem when a gesture "confirms" the patient's statements, or the doctor's hypothesis based on them. Consider this example, in which a patient is suffering from headaches. The physician learns that the patient has been under much stress recently.

Dr: So you have a lot of things on your mind.
Pt: Yes. About them, about some of the members of my family, and, um, mostly it's money worries, mainly money.
Dr: It's funny, when you say 'money worries,' you know where you point to?
Pt: Hah?

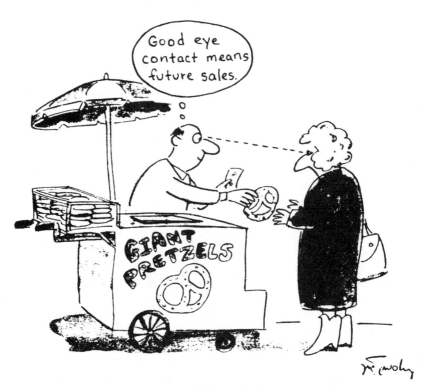

Drawing by M. Twohy; © 1984
The New Yorker Magazine, Inc.

Dr: You point right where it's hurting.
Pt: Yeah, ah hah . . . That's mostly it, you know?

This type of interpretation (in this example, that financial stress may be causing tension headaches) can be very effective both in demonstrating your empathic understanding and in making more explicit a connection the patient may already experience implicitly.

Here are some examples of possible "interpretations" of various gestures (Rakel, 1977). "Steepling" of hands involves joining them with fingers extended and fingertips touching, like a church steeple. Frequently, this indicates confidence or assurance of what is being said. Slight raising of the hand or index finger, pulling at an earlobe, or raising the index finger to the lips, all may indicate a desire to interrupt the speaker. Raising a finger to the lips may also indicate an attempt to suppress a comment.

Crossed arms can be a defensive gesture (indicating disagreement), a sign of insecurity, or simply a comfortable position. Note the manner in which the arms are crossed and the muscular tension, especially in the hands. Fear or tension leads to the "white-knuckle syndrome." Crossed legs may suggest a shutting out of, or protection against, what is going on in the interview, or it may be simply a position of comfort. Uncrossing of the legs while shifting forward in the chair is likely to indicate that the patient is receptive to what you are saying.

Two particular gestures deserve comment. **First** is the helplessness/hopelessness gesture. This is a typically biphasic hand gesture. Both hands are raised briskly to face level, with elbows fixed, palms facing each other rotated slightly outward, fingers spread, and thumb and fingers slightly flexed as though preparing to grasp. This position is held for a second or less, and then the hands fall limply down to the lap. Incomplete variations may be seen. This gesture suggests that the patient feels helpless about the problem or situation. The first part is a reaching out for assistance, while the second part (hypotonia and withdrawal) emphasizes the futility of any help at the moment (Engel, 1977).

The **second** gesture is called the respiratory avoidance response (RAR). This pattern includes frequent clearing of the throat when no phlegm or mucus is present. A variation of this is the nose rub: a light rub of the nose with the dorsal aspect of the index finger. These indicate rejection or disagreement with statements being made. For example, you ask "How are things at home?" The patient answers "Fine," clears his throat, and lightly rubs his nose. He may actually be saying, "I'm uncomfortable with my response; things aren't really going very well at home."

Paralinguistics

When you hear speech, you don't hear just words; you hear words plus pauses. You hear tone of voice and modulation, in addition to specific content. You notice when the patient pauses in his or her story or before answering a question. The functions of pausing include (1) absolute recall time, (2) language formation time, (3) censorship of material, (4) creating an "effect" (timing), and (5) preparing to lie.

People rarely need to pause before recalling a place, age, or date fixed in time. For example, a person readily remembers the age at which a parent died but might have to think a moment before remembering a living parent's current age. It is easy to answer a "yes/no" question without pausing, even if giving the incorrect answer: Do you drink alcohol? Yes. No. This has little meaning. How much alcohol do you usually drink in a day? That question demands some thought and integration. Listen carefully to the answer. How much pause is there? How much stumbling or backtracking? In general, it is helpful to listen to the number, quality, and placement of pauses. Frequent long pauses associated with low amplitude and a "dead" tone suggest depression. Frequent pauses over factual answers throughout the history suggest organic brain dysfunction. Pauses over answers in selected areas may indicate sensitive topics, with time required for censorship of material.

CHAPTER 3

The Medical History, Part 1: Getting Started and the Present Illness

> "Never mind," said Holmes, laughing; "it is my business to know things. Perhaps I have trained myself to see what others overlook. If not, why should you come to consult me?"
>
> Sherlock Holmes, in "A Case of Identity"
> from *Adventures of Sherlock Holmes*

In the next four chapters we discuss, in turn, the traditional parts of a complete medical history—the chief complaint, present illness, past medical history, family history, social history, patient profile, and review of systems. In each section we introduce, describe, and illustrate specific skills or techniques useful for that part of the interview—skills particularly appropriate to its content or medical objective (for example, the review of systems requires a different approach than the history of the present illness). This division of the interview is for simplicity only and does not imply that open-ended questions or interchangeable responses, for example, are useful only in the present illness section. This chapter deals with (1) the setting and how to start, (2) the chief complaint, and (3) explication of the present illness.

STARTING

The Setting

The **setting** for many interviews is often a hospital room. It is important to know how to use that environment to enhance the communication between you and the patient. The hospital is not the patient's natural habitat; as a result, the patient, who is **dis**-eased, may not feel **at** ease. Patients will be similarly uncomfortable, although perhaps less so, in the clinic or doctor's office. When you see a new patient, his blood pressure and pulse will often be elevated, his face flushed, his handshake cool and damp, his gestures clearly nervous. All these indicate the autonomic response to stress—the stress of illness, of seeking help, of meeting a new doctor, of the unknown procedures and outcome. If you appear hurried, indifferent, or unsympathetic, the patient may feel even more uncomfortable; this creates a barrier to effective communication and decreases the accuracy of the data you obtain.

The beginning of the interview sets the atmosphere for the rest of your history and physical examination. This time should be used to establish rapport, demonstrate interest in the patient as a person, and thereby create a base for effective communication. This need not (and should not) take a great deal of time, but it can set the patient at ease. A good history depends as much (or more) on how you ask the questions and the **process** of the interview as on knowing enough pathophysiology to ask the "right" questions.

Establish a sense of **privacy** for the interview. For example, if there is another patient sharing the hospital room, draw the curtain around the bed. While this obviously does not provide a soundproof barrier, it provides the patient with a psychologic sense of privacy. If the patient can walk comfortably, it may be better to interview him or her in a convenient lounge or waiting area, if this will be more private. If the patient has visitors, you might suggest that they wait outside or, if possible, that you will return later to see the patient. Before beginning the history, check to see that the patient is as **comfortable** as possible. Try to seat yourself in a way that will facilitate communication. People have spheres of "personal space" around them: get close enough for a person-to-person interaction, but do not intrude on the patient's intimate space.

In a small hospital room, it may be difficult to place yourself comfortably so that you strike a balance between being halfway across the room and sitting on top of the patient. If necessary, move the chair around. Try to sit at the same level as the patient; this helps establish good eye contact during the interview. Often it is most comfortable to sit at an angle to the person, rather than facing him or her directly; this allows one to maintain good eye contact but also provides natural opportunities to look away at times. Good eye contact does not mean staring fixedly at the patient, which will only make him or her feel uncomfortable; there are always natural breaks in eye contact. You can also use your body to demonstrate interest: by leaning slightly toward the patient, rather than lounging back in your chair, you convey a sense of involvement with what he or she is saying.

How To Start

As you begin the interview, consider these guidelines. **First,** introduce yourself and explain your role. If you are a medical student, introduce yourself as such, or as a "student doctor." Besides being genuine and not using the façade of "doctor" or "consultant," you will also be defining your contract with the patient. As Kimball described, the doctor and patient establish a contract in the interview, albeit usually an unspoken one (Kimball, 1969). The patient expects to describe a complaint and then to have the doctor treat it. If you are a student who does not have responsibility to care for the patient, the contract is limited. When, in the course of the interview, the patient asks your opinion about his or her diagnosis or treatment, asks for pain medication, or requests anything beyond your capacity to respond, you can comfortably remind the patient of the boundaries of your contract. You can tell the patient that you will convey the question or concern to the medical resident or nursing staff, or suggest that the patient do so.

Second, one does not begin by telling the patient, "I've been asked (or sent) to take a history and do a physical." Such a statement is likely to make the patient feel that you have no real interest in him or her, and it may set the interview off on the wrong track. Although it may be true that you are not interviewing the patient on your own initiative, a better start would be "I'd like to talk to you today in order to get some information about why you're in the hospital, and then to examine you." As part of this introduction, you should make certain to obtain permission to do the history and examination; by so doing, you demonstrate interest in and respect for the person.

Third, taking notes is essential, because you will be writing up the information you obtain. As you begin the interview, inform the patient of your need to take notes and the reason; this will also let him or her know what will happen to the information you are obtaining. However, try not to let your note-taking control the interview. If you attempt to record what your patient is saying verbatim (with the exception of the chief complaint), the patient is likely to feel that he or she is being interrogated rather than being interviewed. Eye contact is severely limited if one is mainly concerned with recording the data, and one is likely to miss the patient's nonverbal communication, thereby causing difficulty establishing rapport and missing useful data about the person. While you are making notes during the interview, look up frequently; this will demonstrate interest in the person and in what he or she is saying. One finds with more experience that only an occasional word or phrase need be written down to help one remember, synthesize, and later reconstruct the story.

THE CHIEF COMPLAINT

The **chief complaint** in a standard medical history is the main reason the patient sought medical help, stated in the patient's own words. It is usually recorded verbatim. The chief complaint is often elicited by such questions as:

1. How can I help you today?
2. Can you tell me about your trouble?
3. What symptoms made you decide to see a doctor?
4. Tell me about your problem.
5. Tell me about the main thing you feel is wrong.
6. What brought you to the hospital? (Although this question may be subject to concrete answers like, "A taxi.")

Consider this example of how one medical resident began an interview with a new patient:

Dr: I guess the best place to start is to ask you what brings you here today.

Pt: Well, I haven't had a physical really since six years ago, since my daughter was born.

Dr: I am going to be writing some things down on paper here, okay? Is there any particular reason why you chose now to come in?

Pt: I figured I kept putting it off and putting it off. I'd make appointments and put them off. There was no particular reason. I just felt as though it was time I suppose.

Dr: Nothing is bothering you at this point?

Pt: No, it's just that I am overweight, that's all. I go up and down, up and down.

Dr: So that was your major concern, the weight problem?

Pt: Yeah.

Dr: Can you tell me about that?

The chief complaint here is the weight problem or, stated verbatim, "it's just that I am overweight." It took a little digging to clarify that; we see that the doctor was not satisfied with "there was no particular reason." Sometimes an opening question leads to a clear-cut chief complaint, as in the next example:

Dr: What can I do for you?

Pt: Um, the reason why I'm here is, in the latter part of July up to now, my bowels wouldn't move and I'd have to, in like four and five days, I'd have to take either milk of magnesia or a bulk laxative, and I just thought it was maybe something that I was eating, and this still continues until now and its the reason why I'm here to see you.

In other cases, the same opening question might lead to a much more complex and rambling answer:

Dr: Now what can I do for you, Mrs. P?

Pt: Well, first of all, I'm here mainly because I've been experiencing that tired, worn-out feeling, most of the time. I can go to bed say 9:00 in the evening and get up at 8:00 or even later and I still feel very tired. And, I don't know . . . I've been still experiencing hot flashes and sometimes now . . . I don't experience them as often as I used to but I still do and especially towards the evening or at night, and it awakens me when I do experience something like that. Maybe that's part of the reason why I feel so tired, I don't know. Anyways, now in the evening when I experience this kind of hot feeling I just get that craving I want to eat, you know, or sometimes it works just the opposite where I feel kind of nervous, I get that nervous feeling, and now last week I had headaches just about every day on arising, I had a little runny nose so maybe, I don't know, maybe I could attribute that to a cold, but I'm just mentioning those things to you. And, sometimes you know my head just feels as though, it feels stuffed . . . when you have a head cold, that's just the way it has felt many times, and I had a hysterectomy, let's see, about 1975 or 76 and since then I just have had no sexual desire or anything, I mean as far as I'm concerned that doesn't mean a whole lot. I know it upsets my husband a bit.

What is the chief complaint? Ostensibly, it is her first statement, "mainly because (of) that tired, worn-out feeling . . ." but in context, the situation is less clear. What is really bothering her most? Why did she come here today, as opposed to last month or last week? This particular patient rambles on and on, presenting a type of difficult situation we will discuss in Chapter 8. It is not just the rambling or discursive patient, however, who presents problems in identifying the real chief complaint; often, the actual reason the person comes to see the doctor lies embedded somewhere else, far from his or her initial statement. Here is an example of a patient who presents with chest pain, which he has had for some time:

Dr: I'm glad you came in today. Tell me why you came in.

Pt: Okay. I been having some problems with my chest, you know it's, it's like pressure and plus I have a knot under my arm, under my armpit.

Dr: Okay. You have pressure.

Pt: Yeah, I have pressure and I don't know if it's because I smoke a lot of cigarettes or I don't know what it is.

Dr: Um humm.

Pt: All I know is it's pressure across my chest. It's not what you call a pain or anything, it hurts, it's pressure all across here.

Dr: Um humm.

Pt: And, then, I have this knot under my, under my armpit.

Dr: Okay.

Pt: About the size of a half dollar.

Dr: Okay, let's talk about the chest pain first, when would you say it started?

Pt: Umm, I say about a month ago maybe it might of been longer but I didn't pay it any attention.

Dr: Um hmm.

Pt: You know but I can't jog because if I just start jogging, it bothers me in my chest.

Dr: What made you decide to get it checked?

Pt: Well, two things actually, I want to get back in shape and I got a note from the Health Department that this test came back positive. See, I'm a barber and they test for tuberculosis.

This physician, by asking "What made you decide to get it checked?" not only has the answer to "why now" but an important new piece of data has emerged, namely the positive tuberculin test. We also learn that the patient may believe there is a relationship between his symptoms and the positive test. He really came to the doctor because of the positive tuberculin test, perhaps simply to fulfill a legal requirement for his license and perhaps, in addition, because the positive test made him reinterpret his chest problems as being more serious than they first seemed to be. In any case, if he has no active pulmonary disease the physician knows he will need reassurance that the cause of his trouble lies not in the positive tuberculin test.

When you consider why a person might come for medical help at a certain time, it is not enough simply to elicit a certain symptom or symptoms. The symptoms may have been present for some time. While the answer to these first questions (the chief complaint) frequently contains the core of the patient's problem, sometimes it does not. The **ostensible reason for coming**, as initially stated by the patient in the chief complaint, may not be the same as the **actual reason for coming** (Bass and Cohen, 1982). This is most often true with (1) people who have chronic diseases; (2) people with vague, chronic, and/or recurring symptoms; and (3) people who say they just want a "check-up."

Alvan Feinstein used the term **iatrotropic stimulus** (bringing toward the doctor) to indicate why the patient decided to seek care at this point in time, rather than yesterday, tomorrow, or last year (Feinstein, 1967). The iatrotropic stimulus or the actual reason for coming may be of great importance and not immediately evident. If you can answer the question "Why now?" you have probably uncovered the iatrotropic stimulus or actual reason for coming. Despite the fact that the person has an "acceptable" symptom or disease (heart failure, shortness of breath), it may not satisfactorily explain the whole picture, including why the person sought help today as opposed to last month.

Patients seek care at a certain point in time for different reasons. **First,** the symptoms of the illness may increase to the point when they become unbearable and the person simply realizes he or she needs medical help. We usually assume this one, and often it is quite true in the hospitalized group of patients with whom you have your first interviewing experiences. **Second,** anxiety about the meaning of the symptoms may, for one reason or another, reach the point when the person seeks medical help in spite of the fact that they have been sick for a while or even have **decreasing** symptoms. Perhaps a television news story about a certain disease or the recent diagnosis of a brain tumor in a friend increases the anxiety about an otherwise trivial symptom. **Third,** the symptom in the "chief complaint" may be a "ticket of admission" (Greco and Pittenger, 1966; Balint, 1972) to the doctor's office or hospital; the actual problem may be an entirely different symptom that the patient is at first afraid to mention, or may be some life stress or crisis. If you really listen, the iatrotropic stimulus will come out during the interview. Sometimes it arrives only at the last moment, when you are about to walk out of the room and the patient says, "Oh, by the way, Doc, I'm sure this has nothing to do with it, but . . ." You can prevent this "doorknob phenomenon" by being open-ended and empathic in the beginning; the earlier in the interview you ascertain the patient's reason for coming now, the more efficient you are, wasting less time "digging" for data. Not only will the data be more accurate but so will the diagnosis.

THE PRESENT ILLNESS

The **present illness** is a thorough elaboration of the chief complaint and other current symptoms starting from the time the patient last felt "well" until the present. The best strategy is often, first, to let the patient talk, then to use a variety of nondirective and directive questions to clarify and embellish, generally moving from open-ended questions to more specific "WH" questions, laundry list (menu), or closed-ended questions, as appropriate.

Some examples of **open-ended questions** are:

1. Can you tell me more about that?
2. Did you notice anything else?
3. What was the pain like to you?

Nondirective, or open-ended, questions are always a good way to start, allowing the patient freedom to talk and the examiner time to sit back and "size up" the patient. They are especially good for the less-structured data of the present illness and for psychosocial aspects of the patient's problem, because they allow the patient (who, after all, is the one who "knows") to choose the most important symptoms and to point the way as you develop your interview strategy. The most nondirective of all statements are **minimal facilitators**, queries like (1) "Yes?" (2) "Un huh?" (3) "And?" or (4) "And what else?" Nonverbal cues, such as shaking your head in agreement or smiling, may also serve as minimal encouragers for the patient to continue talking.

After the first few minutes you will have some idea where the interview is going, and you can narrow down the range of open-ended questions by specifying the topics you want to hear more about:

1. Can you tell me more about the **pain**?
2. Do you have any other **medical** problems?

The first indicates you do not want to hear about the shortness of breath just now; the second that you do not want to hear (although perhaps you should) about family or financial problems.

Nondirective questioning, however, usually just sketches the picture, without giving precise detail. Patients only rarely spontaneously volunteer all the needed details; a rambling, vague patient may take too much time and still not give all you need; a shy, reticent patient may say little or nothing. So in a medical interview we move from general to more specific questions. In so doing, it is useful to characterize symptoms by what are called "**WH**" questions (who, what, when, where, why, and how). These describe the attributes of the patient's symptoms and, as Eric Cassell puts it, create a picture of the "disease process marching through the body" (Cassell, 1979). The WH questions are important tools in developing objectivity and precision in the story.

Where: Exactly where is it on your body?

What: What does it feel like?

When: When does it occur (episodic, inception and duration, fluctuation, frequency)?

How: How is it altered by season, by time of day, by sleep, by food, by exertion, and so forth?

Why: Why does it occur? What provokes it? And also, why do you think you have it?

Who: Who is affected by it (consequences to patient and other people)?

Several other kinds of direct questions can be employed as well. **Laundry list questions**, or **menus**, are sometimes useful when a patient cannot find words to express a certain characteristic. For example, "How would you describe this pain—sharp, dull, burning, or tight?" "Would you say it lasted a few seconds, a minute, 10 minutes?" Such questions obviously exclude other descriptive words and are used only when a nondirective approach ("Can you describe the pain?") and "WH" questions ("What is the pain like?") have both failed.

Directive, or **closed-ended**, **questions** provide detail; they are good for emergency situations ("What's your name?" "How old are you?" "Are you allergic to any drugs?"), reticent patients, and for structured historic data, such as the past history and the review of systems. However, a "high-control" interview in which the interviewer asks one directive question after another, will produce false or incomplete evidence, not to mention a discontented patient. Some examples of closed-ended questions are:

1. Are your parents still living?
2. Did you pass out?
3. Have you ever been anemic?

This type of yes/no question gives only minimal information, but this is all you need for certain cut-and-dried parts of the history: "Is your father alive?" "Do you have any allergies?" "Is there any trouble with your vision?" Such questions are most useful for screening-type questions, as in the review of systems. One does not ask **yes/no questions** in situations when information may be sensitive, because a lie will close off all access to that information. For example, it is not useful to say "Do you drink alcohol?" if one suspects alcohol may be a problem; try, "How much alcohol do you usually drink in a day?"

Finally, one avoids **leading questions**, which encourage certain responses from the patient to fit the interviewer's own hypothesis, such as "You're feeling better now, aren't you?" or "That pain wasn't on the left side of your chest, was it?" This type of query suggests to the patient what you want (or don't want) to hear. Likewise, one avoids **multiple questions**, such as: "Do you have any trouble sleeping, how about cough?" Sometimes these slip out, because your mind is working too quickly and dragging your tongue along with it. Slow down, wait. Table 2 summarizes these various types of queries employed in the medical history.

Symptom Description

Throughout the history of the present illness, it is important to describe the patient's symptoms as carefully as possible without jumping to conclusions. For example, "I'm short of breath" is not necessarily "dyspnea on

TABLE 2. Types of Questions in Medical History Taking

Start with	Open-ended questions: General
	Minimal facilitators
	Open-ended questions: Topic
Then proceed to	"WH" questions
	Laundry lists or menus
	Direct questions
	Yes/No questions
Avoid	Leading questions
	Complex or multiple questions

exertion" or "orthopnea;" you need more details. It is also important to avoid jumping to conclusions about the meanings of certain words. Many words commonly used to describe symptoms mean different things to different people. Some examples are diarrhea, constipation, tired, dizzy, "my side," sick, weak, high blood, low blood, insomnia, gas, and heartburn. The novice has a tendency to establish quantitative ("How many times a day?") aspects of symptoms before establishing the qualitative. The expert interviewer attempts to establish what he or she is dealing with ("Are the stools soft or watery?") before measuring it. One wants to establish the picture, the pattern, how things hang together, the **gestalt;** then one fills in the quantitative data. Table 3 presents some examples of patient statements, followed by either **quantitative** (prematurely specific) or **qualitative** physician follow-up questions.

It is important not to get caught up in the "New Brunswick syndrome" when taking the patient's history. A friend of ours was living in Canada and his mother from New Jersey was visiting. They were invited to a party and our friend noted that his mother was carrying on a long, animated discussion with a woman with whom he thought she had nothing in com-

TABLE 3. Patient Complaints and Possible Quantitative or Qualitative Physician Questions

Complaint	Quantitative Questions	Qualitative Questions
I've been having chest pain.	How long have you had it? How often does it come?	What does it feel like? Where exactly is it located?
My side hurts.	How long have you had it?	Show me where.
I have diarrhea.	How many times a day?	What do you mean by diarrhea?
I vomited blood.	How much?	What did it look like?
I can't walk as far as I used to without getting tired.	How far can you walk?	What do you mean by "tired?"

mon. Afterward, he asked his mother what they were talking about. She said, "Well, we were sharing a lot of memories of our childhoods in New Brunswick." They carried on a long, gratifying conversation despite the fact that one was talking about New Brunswick, New Jersey, and the other was referring to the Canadian Province of New Brunswick. The same words mean different things to different people. This does not present too much of a problem at a cocktail party, but it can be deadly in the medical history. This is what we mean by **precision** in obtaining data: we must describe exactly what occurred and not suffer from the "New Brunswick syndrome" of medical words.

The symptom called "dizziness" presents a prime example. A patient comes in and says, "My main problem is dizziness. It just came on me about a month ago, and it's been getting worse now. I'm so dizzy I can hardly stand up sometimes. What's wrong with me, Doc?" The first thing that is wrong is the word "dizziness." According to Reilly (1984), there are at least four common syndromes or symptoms vaguely labeled with this word. These include (1) vertigo, a definite rotational sensation or sense of environmental motion; (2) presyncope, the sensation that loss of consciousness is about to happen; (3) disequilibrium, the sensation that balance, especially during walking, is impaired; and (4) lightheadedness, a vague head sensation that is not vertigo and not presyncope. There are also other symptoms as well, such as weakness, fatigue, or anxiety, that some persons idiosyncratically label as "dizziness."

The following exchange, adapted from Reilly's *Practical Strategies in Outpatient Medicine* (1984, p. 457), shows an example of a doctor trying to find out precisely what a patient means by dizziness:

> Dr: Can you describe what you mean with words other than dizzy?
> Pt: I feel out of balance. I feel like I might fall down even. I haven't yet, but I get awful woozy when I walk.
> Dr: Is it mainly when you walk that you have trouble or do you get this feeling sometimes when you are sitting or resting?
> Pt: I guess it is mainly when I am up and around.
> Dr: Can you tell me, then, how you feel bad when you walk? Try not to say dizzy.
> Pt: Well, I feel I'm unsure of myself. I can't trust my walking.
> Dr: Does everything around you spin or move, or do you feel like you're spinning?
> Pt: No, not exactly.
> Dr: Do you feel like you are going to faint?
> Pt: I feel like I will fall, not faint.

There is much more to find out about this symptom, but from the exchange so far the patient appears to be describing disequilibrium, rather than vertigo, presyncope, or lightheadedness. Another example of the "New Brunswick Syndrome" arose in the following interchange with a patient who came to the doctor because of her cough. Note how the clinician begins with an open-ended question, specifying only that he wishes to hear about the cough, then follows up with the "WH" questions until he knows precisely what the symptom is.

Dr: Tell me about the **cough** that you've been having.
Pt: It's just, worse at night, I can't get no sleep.
Dr: What happens?
Pt: I'm up on three pillows, I'm just miserable that's all.
Dr: You go up on three pillows to try to prevent the cough?
Pt: Yes.
Dr: How is it miserable?
Pt: Well, if I lay flat I can't breathe, and then I start gasping and gasping for breath, and the only way I can stop is when I sit up and watch TV or something.

The patient in this example actually suffered from congestive heart failure with orthopnea; she became short of breath when she lay flat in bed. She experienced a tightness in her chest and a sense of "gasping" for breath which she chose to call "cough." Later in the conversation, the doctor learned that she had anginal chest pain and dyspnea on exertion, as well as these nocturnal symptoms.

In this longer example, the physician wants to pin down the exact timing of the onset, duration, periodicity, and pattern of chest pain. The doctor is concerned that the symptom in this 62-year-old smoker may be caused by coronary artery disease, and knows that only precise symptom description will guide the diagnostic process. Each time the patient gives a somewhat vague statement, the physician follows up with an attempt at clarification (these are preceded by an asterisk).

Pt: . . . and little bit too fast, it might just be my imagination though, I don't know.
Dr: Uh huh. When did this all start?
Pt: Well, just since the weather has been hot, like it is, you know.
*Dr: Several weeks it's been going on, would you say?
Pt: Uh huh, just—now the chest pain is not continuous, like, during the day, I don't have to be doing anything, I can just be sitting.
Dr: And where do you feel it?
Pt: It's in here. And like full, just too full, it's fullness in here.
Dr: And then how long does it last when it comes?
Pt: Not too long.

*Dr: Minutes, hours?

Pt: Not hours, just maybe a half hour, or something—you know, it doesn't last.

*Dr: Do you do anything that seems to relieve it?

Pt: No, I don't take anything, just sit and be quiet, or either I'll rest. Like, the neighbors, like I told you, were throwing out those old chairs—that recliner, I could use it so, he helped me with it, he put it over the fence and helped me with it into the house and that helps a whole lot. I go in and stretch out on that.

Dr: Uh huh.

Pt: And rest seems to help, when it starts acting up, whenever I could or would be doing around the house, let it go and just rest.

*Dr: Does it sometimes come on while you are doing something?

Pt: Yeah, mostly, if I'm doing something like trying to sweep or clean in the house or something like that.

*Dr: How about with walking?

Pt: With walking sometimes, and like mostly. I'll go up to the mall every day and that way I am inside walking and they have benches, I'll sit . . . when it starts acting up.

*Dr: And then how long does it take to go away once you sit?

Pt: Once I sit, oh, I'll say, half an hour to an hour.

*Dr: And it will take a half hour or an hour to go away?

Pt: Uh huh.

*Dr: Or do you sit for that long even though it's gone before that?

Pt: Uh huh. I just sit for that long until it eases.

*Dr: And it takes a half hour to an hour for it to ease up?

Pt: Uh huh.

Dr: Do you have any other symptoms along with it when you have the pain?

Pt: No.

Summaries, Confrontations, Clarifications

A summary is a technique by which the clinician feeds back to the patient the high points of what has been said thus far. Frequent summaries ensure that the interviewer has the story straight, help terminate one area of the history and launch another, and help the interviewer remain organized. A summary may be as simple as repeating a particularly important statement to see if you have it right, such as: "Okay, as I understand it, the pains you had in 1980 were exactly like the ones you're having now . . ." In other cases a brief summary helps one get back on track if the patient is wandering and switching topics: "Okay, we'll get to the cough in a minute, but I need to understand your chest pain better. You said it was like a heavy pressure right in the center of your chest, and it lasted about five minutes . . ."

Summaries are also very useful as transitions from one part of the interview to another. This allows both you and the patient to keep track of where you have been and where you are going. Here is an example of a summary that leads into a transition from the history of the present illness to the past medical history:

Pt: So that's about how it happened.
Dr: Okay, let me see if I have it straight. You felt perfectly well until two days ago when you began to notice an uncomfortable feeling right in the middle here around your belly button, and this has gradually gotten worse and you are now also having diarrhea. *(Patient nods).* Okay, I think I understand pretty well what's been going on the last two days. How about in the past, have you had any problems with your health in the past?

Sometimes as you try to summarize, you note discrepancies in the patient's story; and because you want to know exactly what happened, it is often necessary to point out those discrepancies. When you do this, you are "confronting" the patient. This rather dramatic word arose from interviewing techniques in psychotherapy. It has connotations of pointing out falsehoods, rationalizations, or neurotic conflicts, and in its everyday usage often implies opposing sides. In the medical interview, however, **confrontation** is often simply a request for clarification; you heard one thing and now it appears the patient is describing his experience differently, or contradicting an earlier statement. Which version is right?

Dr: Now let me see if I can understand this. You said before that you were coughing up some bloody stuff with that heavy cough last year. But just now you said, when this cough developed yesterday, it was the first time you ever saw blood come up? Did I misunderstand you?

A **clarification** falls somewhere between a summary and a confrontation. You say what you heard but ask for more detail, perhaps to clear up some discrepancies in the story.

SUMMARY OF FACILITATIVE TECHNIQUES

We now summarize those techniques presented in the first three chapters that help any interviewer obtain accurate and precise data during the initial part of the medical history.

1. Maintain an attentive body position and minimize distractions, achieving a sense of privacy for both you and the patient.
2. Take notes, but maintain enough eye contact so as not to "lose" the patient.
3. Use language the patient can understand. This means translating certain terms as they may appear in an outline of a history or present themselves in your head into words with which the patient is familiar.
4. Structure questions to go from general to specific, using open-ended questions to introduce the history or each part of the history and then proceeding to more specific questioning.
5. Use minimal encouragers or facilitators, such as silence with or without a head nod, but almost always looking at the patient; repeating a key word or the last word before the patient pauses; saying "un huh" or "and?"; saying "and what else?" or "for example?"
6. Proceed to "WH" questions to characterize symptoms.
7. Employ menus or direct questions when necessary for specification or efficiency.
8. Strive for **interchangeable responses** to encourage more information and show that you are listening. This means restating what the patient has said, using a combination of your own words and those of the patient to show you "understand exactly" (see Chapter 2). One way of doing this is through effective use of mirrors and paraphrases. A "mirror" or reflective response is simply feeding back to the patient exactly what he or she said:

> Pt: I feel really terrible.
> Dr: You feel really terrible? *(mirror)*
> **or**
> Dr: You're not feeling so well, huh. *(paraphrase)*

9. Avoid leading questions that reveal the answer you expect or desire, or multiple questions that confuse the patient.
10. Give the patient time to answer in his or her own words. This means waiting a little while and not being afraid to endure silence as you wait.
11. Clarify and maintain direction for both yourself and the patient by using summaries, clarification, and, when needed, confrontation.
12. Feed back positives (for instance, the patient's strengths as you see them) to help develop the relationship, support the patient, and elicit more information. Example:

> Dr: It sounds as though you've been coping really well, despite a lot of pain for some time now. Now let's talk about what happened just yesterday to make things worse . . .

13. Keep a simple "roadmap" in your head (or on a note card) of where you intend to go in the interview, and to remind you of where you are.

EXAMPLES

We conclude this chapter with three examples of beginnings of interviews. In each case, we have labeled the physician's statements or questions with the term that describes the technique being used. Note the importance, in this part of the interview, of social greetings, nondirective questions, clarification, minimal facilitators, and summaries.

Example 1

> Dr: Okay, hello again. I'm Dr. Block. Tell me what I can do for you today. *(social greeting, nondirective question)*
>
> Pt: Well, I have a terrible vaginal itch, and I don't know whether it's the vaginitis or whether it's the urine, urinary tract infection. My regular doctor treated me for vaginitis.
>
> Dr: That was Dr. Hill? *(clarification, facilitation)*
>
> Pt: Uh huh. Then I got, um, a urinary tract infection and then the vaginitis came back. But, during the whole ordeal, I've never got any relief.
>
> Dr: During the treatment for the vaginitis, during the treatment for the urinary tract infection, you still had this terrible itch? *(summary)*

Example 2

> Dr: Good morning. *(social greeting)*
>
> Pt: *(Seated on end of exam table.)* Good morning.
>
> Dr: Why don't you have a seat back over here and we can talk a little bit first. Tell me why you came today. *(seeing to patient's comfort, nondirective question)*
>
> Pt: Um, to get my blood pressure checked.
>
> Dr: To get your blood pressure checked? What do you know about your blood pressure? *(reflective response, nondirective question with topic specified)*

Pt: Well, I have heard various things over the past couple of years, really, that it has been high, and um . . .

Dr: For several years? *(clarification, facilitation)*

Pt: *(Nods)* And I went about, oh, it was quite a while ago, maybe five or six months ago to the health center, um, and the doctor told me it was high and also, but he could not treat me until I lost approximately 38 pounds, so I haven't been able to take the weight off and I was kind of, well, he did not give me any special diet to follow or you know, what I should cut out of my diet, and I was very discouraged by it, so when I went to the emergency room because I cut my finger, um, the nurse told me that my blood pressure was very high and I should have something, you know, checked, and I should have it checked, and since I don't have a family doctor, she suggested I come here.

Example 3

Dr: It's nice to see you again. What brings you here today? *(social greeting, open-ended question)*

Pt: Doctor, I'm not well.

Dr: I take it you have not been feeling really well for a while. *(summary based on previous knowledge of this patient)*

Pt: No, well, I haven't been feeling very good for about the last, oh, I'd say about a week, about a week now.

Dr: Uh huh. *(facilitation)*

Pt: About a week now, I haven't been feeling good.

Dr: What have you noticed? *(nondirective question)*

Pt: Oh, some soreness in here right through here, and some pain in my arm and a, a, a strangulating feeling right in here and a burning in the, in the middle, right here and a burning in my throat, a little bit, and dizzy—I felt real dizzy when I was on the scale out there, you know, and I called you and the nurse, and she helped me and I wasn't real bad and you know, I told her to open a window and she said first 'Do you want me to open a window?' and I said 'Yeah and I want to get near the air.'

Dr: Does that help? *(clarification)*

Pt: Oh yeah.

We now move on to consider the more structured aspects of the medical history.

CHAPTER 4

Medical History, Part 2: The Past History, the Family History, and the Review of Systems

> To hold a true belief about an event in one's past experience is not sufficient for remembering it. There is still a distinctive factor lacking . . . Now it sometimes happens that a belief . . . transforms itself into a memory.
>
> Alfred Jules Ayer, *The Problem of Knowledge*

Once you have elicited the chief complaint, iatrotropic stimulus, and complete description of your patient's present illness, other parts of the history, while tedious at first, are in a sense easier, because they deal with structured data and are specific questions about predetermined topics. The skill lies in being precise about important details, while avoiding overinterpretation of the unimportant; later, you will be able to relate pertinent information from the past medical history or review of systems to your patient's current illness. The trick is to emphasize the relevant features of past health and medical care experiences without getting too overwhelmed with a mass of detail. Alvan Feinstein has taught his students to avoid the "Scylla of Overdirection" and the "Charybdis of Digression." By this he meant the ability to keep the inquiry open-ended enough to avoid missing the important without getting bogged down in endless details about unimportant events.

This chapter and the one following will cover parts of the medical interview that fill in the total picture of your patient's health and illness experience. These aspects of the interview provide important details that enhance your evaluation of and response to the person's current illness. In this chapter we will discuss the past medical history, family history, and review of systems. These components help complete the picture by providing you with information about the context or setting in which the illness occurs, including the previous state of the patient's health as well as the presence of risk factors, which have implications for both current diagnosis and the prevention of future ills. We cover the patient's personal profile or social history in Chapter 5.

THE PAST MEDICAL HISTORY (PMH)

You can begin your inquiry with a quite general question, such as "How has your health been in the past?" Another possibility is "Tell me about any serious illnesses you have had in the past, starting from when you were a child." A third possibility: "Now I'd like to ask you about any illnesses or medical problems you've had in the past. How has your health been?" Or you can provide a transition from the present illness, such as "Okay, I think I understand what's been happening the last few weeks; how about your health in the past?"

Patients may answer in quite general terms, such as "I've always been sickly," or "Well, I used to have stomach problems," or they may begin to discuss particular symptoms. You must try to focus the inquiry on (1) discrete episodes that (2) caused substantial disability or a difference in the usual health pattern, and attempt to determine (3) the name that the patient or patient's doctor has given to these illnesses. You should never simply accept a diagnosis that a patient relates to you as being, in fact, the correct medical diagnosis. This is true even when a patient says she was hospitalized and was told her problem was a "heart attack" or "pneumonia." Many patients will tell you they have had "four or five heart attacks" in the past when, in fact, they have never suffered a documented acute myocardial infarction; this problem arises because their use of the term "heart attack" is not the same as your use of that term. A good question to ask is "What exactly were your symptoms that made the doctor think that?"

There is no point, however, in obsessively trying to confirm every item of the past history by grilling the patient on obscure details. Your time and energy and those of the patient are limited. Consider how asking about "ancient history" is apt to make the patient feel:

> "It's bad enough that I don't know all my family's medical diseases or of what my grandparents, whom I never knew, died, but I begin to feel positively stupid when at the mature age of forty-four I do not know whether as an infant I had measles or chicken pox. I may do a little better with more recent conditions but the feeling sinks again when it comes to medications I've taken that have given me trouble. 'Those little red pills' seem an insufficient answer and the recording physician's dubious look does not help much . . . By this point in the interview when I am asked questions about the specific timing and location of my varying symptoms, I begin to answer with a specificity born more of desperation than accuracy." (Eisenberg and Kleinman, 1980)

Old records can and should be obtained when, on the basis of your complete evaluation, you believe the information will be relevant to caring for the person's present illness, or for their future general medical care.

Many adult patients will have one or more chronic illnesses, and often each of these may have had several exacerbations or required hospitalization at different times. It is necessary to consider the relevance of these to the current illness. Consider the patient who was referred to a medical faculty member because of rapidly progressive congestive heart failure symptoms, who had no clear evidence of ischemic heart disease, and who was not hypertensive. The referring doctor thought the patient might have a congestive cardiomyopathy because of her dilated heart, predominance of severe right-sided heart failure, and symptoms that appeared to begin rather suddenly one year before. However, her past medical history revealed quite frequent episodes of "acute bronchitis" and "pneumonia," and the review of systems also yielded the information that she had a chronic "cigarette" cough, usually producing a fair amount of sputum each morning. She was found to have chronic obstructive pulmonary disease with heart failure on the basis of cor pulmonale. She had not (nor had her physician!) related her recurrent lung problems and cigarette smoking to the illness at hand. When the doctor made this connection, it became clear that the present illness really extended much further into the past than was initially thought to have been the case.

After you acquire general information about the person's past health, you should fill in important categories of past medical history as shown in Table 4.

The exact date or even year, if it is remote, is generally not important. Inquiry that is too precise will lead both to frustration and to answers that are likely to be falsely precise. A "hysterectomy in the early 1960s" is usually adequate; it does not matter whether it was 1962 or 1963. You should try to clarify what your patient means by the term "allergy." A person may tell you he is allergic to flu shots because, after having one, he went on to have several colds that winter; or a person may tell you that she is allergic

TABLE 4. Past Medical History

---

1. Serious illnesses, from childhood through the most recent
2. Hospitalizations for these problems
3. Surgical procedures
4. Accidents or injuries
5. Pregnancies, deliveries, and complications (women)
6. Immunizations
7. Allergies
8. Medications currently used (including over-the-counter drugs and vitamins)

---

to aspirin because it gives her stomach discomfort. The first case is a personal attribution of some poor outcome, while the second case illustrates a side effect rather than a true allergy to aspirin. Be sure to ask specifically about allergies to medications. You should inquire what medications the patient is currently taking (or supposed to take), but also broaden your inquiry to include any regularly used drugs, such as oral contraceptives (which the patient may not consider a "medication"), cold preparations, pain relievers, or laxatives obtained without a prescription. Remember also to ask about vitamins or mineral (for example, iron) tablets, because many people consider these "natural" products and not medication; they may not mention them unless specifically asked.

When you go to do your write-up keep two things in mind: (1) transfer data relevant to the current problem into the history of the present illness; and (2) make liberal use of quotation marks to indicate what the patient says that you have not actually confirmed such as "hysterectomy," "allergy," or "slipped disc."

Here is an example of a past medical history obtained from a 39-year-old woman at her first office visit for evaluation of headaches. She was found to have an elevated blood pressure.

Dr: Okay, let's talk about your past health. Did you have any unusual childhood illnesses, rheumatic fever, scarlet fever, diphtheria?

Pt: Bronchitis.

Dr: Bronchitis. What do you mean by bronchitis?

Pt: Well, I'm not sure. That's what my mother told me. I guess I used to get sick a lot when I was a kid.

Dr: Were you ever hospitalized? Any serious illnesses or operations?

Pt: Uh huh.

Dr: What have you been hospitalized for?

Pt: When I've had D and Cs done and I had my appendix out with part of my ovary.

Dr: Part of your ovary came out and . . . ?

Pt: Well, I have a history of cysts growing on my ovaries.

Dr: Were you followed by a gynecologist?

Pt: Yes, Dr. Smith here in town.

Dr: Now, you mentioned you have two children. Any problems with your pregnancies or with childbirth?

Pt: With my little girl, yes. I had a lot of water, plus I had a bladder infection.

Dr: Did you have high blood pressure with that?

Pt: No, but I was sick a lot, nauseated a lot. It was like morning sickness but I had it for eight months with her.

Dr: Doctor put you to bed at all?

Pt: No.

Dr: Any other hospitalizations, any other medical problems in the past that you had that you can remember?

Pt: No, just the D and Cs and the children and that one operation I had.

Dr: Do you have any known allergies?

Pt: I am allergic to goldenrod.

Dr: To what?

Pt: Goldenrod. Wool. I have hay fever. Anything like flowers—I get around them, I constantly sneeze my head off or get stuffed up. Roses, stuff like that. Right now, I'm having a time because we went up to the lake and we have a lot of goldenrod growing wild.

Dr: Do you take anything for it?

This is an example of a fairly typical and complete past history that maintains its relevance to the problems at hand. Notice how the physician asks exactly what the patient means by "bronchitis." Although the patient is not sure, she later reports symptoms of allergy; symptoms of allergy plus a childhood history of "bronchitis" suggest atopy, with the "bronchitis" perhaps representing episodes of childhood asthma. The patient has now "outgrown" her asthma but still has an atopic disposition as evidenced by the hayfever symptoms. The physician also uncovers the history of fluid retention during pregnancy. This could have been a sign of toxemia, possibly of relevance to her hypertension now. Notice how he asks specifically if the patient had high blood pressure; he also asks for the information in another way ("Doctor put you to bed at all?"), as this action might indicate an increased blood pressure with the physician not so informing the patient. Another way to ask this (especially if you have no idea what the therapy might have been) would be, "How was that treated?" The question regarding whether the patient takes anything for her hayfever is relevant on at least three counts: (1) the physician can avoid the embarrassment of recommending something the patient has already tried; (2) knowledge of what the patient has tried and how successful treatment proved indicates something of the severity of the symptoms; and (3) some decongestants will raise the blood pressure in susceptible individuals or when used to excess.

Here is another example, a simpler past history. Notice how the physician starts with a general question ("What other medical problems have you had?"), then focuses in on specific illnesses and finally surgeries:

Dr: What other medical problems have you had?

Pt: None.

Dr: Has anyone ever told you that your blood pressure was high?

Pt: No.
Dr: Have you ever had a problem with sugar diabetes?
Pt: No.
Dr: Okay, what medications are you presently taking?
Pt: Just the Urecholine.
Dr: How much do you take?
Pt: About four times a day.
Dr: No other medications?
Pt: No.
Dr: Okay, what other surgery have you had in the past?
Pt: My appendix.
Dr: What year was that?
Pt: 1979, I think 1980.
Dr: Did your appendix rupture?
Pt: Uh huh.
Dr: It did rupture. Any other surgery?
Pt: No. My tonsils.
Dr: Your tonsils as a child?
Pt: Yeah.

Our final example is that of a patient who was being seen for back pain and reported a past history of phlebitis. What follows is the physician's search for the evidence (in how the patient was diagnosed and treated) that she did, indeed, have phlebitis:

Pt: But I have more trouble in my left leg than I do in the right leg, normally with this phlebitis that I had.
Dr: Did you ever have, were you ever admitted to the hospital for phlebitis and given intravenous medicines?
Pt: It's so long ago I don't remember.
Dr: Did you ever take a blood thinner?
Pt: Yes, Coumadin.
Dr: You were on Coumadin at one time. Did they ever do any x-ray studies of your legs with a dye. Did they ever put a . . .
Pt: I had the fibrinogen test. I had a series of tests.
Dr: Fibrinogen scans . . .
Pt: Yes, I had a series of tests done.
Dr: Did they ever do a venogram?
Pt: I don't know what that is.
Dr: You would remember it, a venogram is where they put a needle into a vein in your foot and they inject a dye.
Pt: No, they didn't do that.
Dr: So you haven't had a venogram done.
Pt: I was taking iodine and had to take the iodine every day and

come to the hospital every day for a month. I think that was the fibrinogen test.

Dr: The fibrinogen scan. Did you ever have, I imagine you would have had something called a Doppler study.

Pt: I don't remember.

Dr: Or IPG, that's where they use sound waves to look for clots in the legs.

Pt: Is it a machine?

Dr: Yes.

Pt: I was on a machine in the emergency room one night.

Dr: On a machine for . . .

Pt: . . . for phlebitis.

Dr: Checking your legs, or do you mean one of the IV machines?

Pt: No, it wasn't IV.

Dr: Is it a machine where they ran a little microphone like thing?

Pt: No, they put little things on like they're going to take your blood pressure. They put them on my legs.

Dr: So they were studying blood clots. So, you have been on . . . were you only on the Coumadin one time?

Pt: Twice.

Dr: Twice. And you were hospitalized both times?

Pt: No, I wasn't hospitalized.

Dr: You weren't. You were never hospitalized before you were put on Coumadin.

Pt: No. I was in the emergency room and then I went to the doctor's office.

Dr: And they put you on Coumadin. You never had any heparin.

Pt: No, I didn't have heparin. I had Coumadin. The little white pills.

Dr: Right. That's interesting.

THE FAMILY HISTORY

The **family history** is the systematic exploration of the presence or absence of any illness in the patient's family that may have an impact on the diagnosis of the present illness or on other concurrent illnesses, or that influences the patient's health or risk of future disease. This simple statement obscures the important questions: (1) what "illnesses" are relevant? and (2) what do we mean by "family?"

First, what illnesses and conditions are relevant? Relevant illnesses include (1) frankly hereditary diseases, such as sickle cell anemia or dyslipoproteinemias; (2) "familial" illnesses, such as coronary artery disease, adult-onset diabetes mellitus, or carcinoma of the breast, in which the genetic transmission is not as clear cut but in which familial clustering may become manifest in the presence of appropriate environmental stimuli; (3) family "traits," such as short stature; (4) illnesses such as schizophrenia or alcoholism, which not only may be familial but also may profoundly affect the patient's past and present environments; and (5) current illnesses that suggest a common infectious or toxic exposure among family members.

Second, by "family" we generally mean (for familial/hereditary disease) the patient's parents, siblings, and children (of first importance) and the patient's grandparents, cousins, aunts, and uncles (of somewhat lesser importance). The spouse is a vital member of the patient's family but is of no importance to familial disease. Sometimes we must distinguish "family" from "household," as when the interviewer is considering environmental (toxic exposure) or contagious illness, perhaps even broadening the definition to include the patient's place of work.

The family history always enriches our understanding of the patient, whether in "getting" the diagnosis or in managing the illness; but because time and energy are limited, the potentially enormous amount of information must be tailored to the specific situation. How much one wants to know depends on the patient and the illness—the acuteness of the illness, age and sex of the patient, type of problem, and the ability of the patient to give the information. For example, a family history of breast cancer is of less relevance to a 10-year-old boy with tonsillitis than to a 45-year-old woman with a breast mass. A seriously ill patient may have a very relevant family history but be too sick to give any but the most critical data about the recent progression of symptoms. This might be the situation, say, in a patient with an acute myocardial infarction who has a strong family history of coronary artery disease; if there is no ambiguity about the diagnosis, the family history can wait until the patient feels well enough to remember and discuss the details. And these details will be vital as the patient recovers, because how he feels about his future will be colored by his recollections and beliefs about family members who had or have the same diagnosis.

A good way to start with the routine family history is "Are there any illnesses that seem to run in your family?" or "Has anyone in your family been seriously ill? How about your parents? Children?" It is almost always helpful to ask "Has anyone in your family ever had anything like the symptoms you are having now?" Or, if you know the diagnosis, "Has anyone in your family had heart attacks?" In the case of an acute, possibly contagious illness, a helpful question to begin with is "Has anyone else at home or work been sick lately?" or "Have you come into contact with anyone who has similar symptoms?"

Here is an excerpt of a routine family history that will give you some sense of the flow of this part of the medical interview. Notice how the physician first introduces the new subject area (a transition), and then goes on with a specific question:

> Dr: Okay, I think I understand the symptoms. Now I'd like to find out a little about your family. How about your parents, are they still living?
> Pt: They're deceased.
> Dr: Do you recall what they passed away from?
> Pt: My mother had a heart attack two months ago.
> Dr: How old was she at that time?
> Pt: Sixty-three, I think.
> Dr: How about your father?
> Pt: About seven years ago.
> Dr: What did he pass away from?
> Pt: Lung cancer.
> Dr: How old was he?
> Pt: Oh, I'd say 57.
> Dr: Brothers or sisters?
> Pt: Yes, I have nine brothers—I mean I have five brothers and three sisters.
> Dr: Do they have medical problems that you are aware of?
> Pt: No.
> Dr: Is there any history of high blood pressure in the family?
> Pt: My mother.
> Dr: Your mother, okay. How about diabetes?
> Pt: No.

The physician begins with a general question asking first about problems or illnesses, then follows up with some very specific yes/no questions about illnesses that one tends to see in families (such as hypertension and diabetes) or illnesses of particular relevance to this patient (who has hypertension).

But we observe something else here. There is no way to avoid the fact that some of the information we obtain is at once medical and social. Because the "family" is a social unit, the information we obtain in this part of the history invariably has some "social" aspects to it. The fact of the matter is that the information we seek in the family history is almost never neutral information: everyone has feelings about his or her close relatives, especially parents and children. There is no way to avoid this; we can, however, acknowledge it, be prepared for it, and deal with it in a compassionate way during the interview.

In the previous example, notice that the patient's mother is very recently deceased. This is certainly not emotionally neutral information. The physician here faces a choice about how to proceed, whether or not to explore the patient's feelings, simply to make an empathic statement, or to continue getting information. In this instance, the doctor continues to get more information and this appears to be useful. Had the patient's mother died in old age after increasing illness or disability, the physician would expect the patient to have different feelings than if she died suddenly at a relatively young age. A potential problem here is that the physician takes his patient's word for "heart attack" and learns little more. There are many possibilities: Was it sudden? After many previous attacks? Was she sickly for years, perhaps with rheumatic heart disease, and suffered a final "attack"? And what of the resulting effects on a patient with a sickly mother?

What the patient "knows" about his or her family shapes his or her beliefs and worries about his or her health, health risks, and current symptoms. A patient with chest pain may believe that she has a bad heart like her mother, even though she is young and suffering from a totally different type of problem. A patient approaching the same age as that at which a parent died may have special concerns about his or her own health. Consider this family history in a 41-year-old woman who came because "it's been a while since I had a good check-up":

> Dr: Your parents still living?
> Pt: My father is living. My mother died when she was 42.
> Dr: How is your father? Is he in good health?
> Pt: Uh huh.
> Dr: How old is he?
> Pt: He was born in 1919.
> Dr: So he's 67.
> Pt: Yes.
> Dr: Any brothers or sisters.
> Pt: Two sisters. Both are in good health as far as I know. I don't keep very good contact with them, because I live here and they live out of state.
> Dr: Any medical problems? You said there are some medical problems that run in your family. What are they again?
> Pt: My mother had a bad heart. Most of it is in my mother's family. Like my grandmother died, she had cancer. She had diabetes too. When my mother died she had a plastic valve put in, then slowly deteriorated. She had sclerosis of the liver and a bad heart. She lived about a year after she had the plastic valve put in.

Again, this information is two-sided; a woman who dies at the age of 42 after having an artificial valve, probably had rheumatic (or possibly congenital) heart disease. While there is some chance that the daughter may suffer from a similar problem, of more relevance is whether the daughter believes herself to be at risk. If she is found to have no signs of heart disease, it will be important to reassure her that her symptoms are totally unrelated to what went on with her mother.

Even the most straightforward questions tend to produce double-edged information:

> Dr: You said you've been pregnant five times?
> Pt: Yes.
> Dr: Do your children live at home with you?
> Pt: Yes.
> Dr: Five of them?
> Pt: Yes.
> Dr: How old are they?
> Pt: 20, 15, 13, 10.
> Dr: That's four children.
> Pt: Oh, I lost one.
> Dr: Did he die of a disease?
> Pt: No, he died—he had a little growth on his eye and he died in surgery.

The physician dedicated to a mechanical set of questions for family history could have simply ignored the fact she only gave four ages. While the death of her child seems to have no strictly "medical" bearing whatever, a parent who has lost a child will certainly have feelings attached to the memory of the event.

Yet another problem in doing the family history is that while you wish to raise awareness or simply obtain neutral information, you may increase anxiety. In the asking about family diseases, whether or not they are frankly hereditary, there is an implicit statement that the history matters to the patient's medical problem now. It is helpful to be reassuring about this and to emphasize the "routine" nature of the inquiry. If you do not know whether there is a connection between the patient's family history and his or her present illness, say that you do not know but explore how the patient would feel if there were a connection. Do not raise anxiety unnecessarily. Here is an example of a physician who stumbles on anxiety-provoking information in asking a routine family history question:

> Dr: Yeah, okay. Very good. Now your mother and father, what did they . . . Are they still alive?
> Pt: Um, my mother is alive, my . . .
> Dr: Age?

Notice how the physician hesitates over the initial question, realizing that the first thing he needs to know is if the parents are living, then barely listening to the response, he asks his next question. The dialogue continues:

Pt: She is 64.
Dr: She have any illnesses you know of?
Pt: Uh . . .
Dr: Heart disease, lung disease, anything?
Pt: No, nothing of that sort, she's had a well-known skin cancer and uh, and she seems to have a recurring, it's a problem with her back, but actually it's a nerve that has to be blocked every once in a while.
Dr: Okay. Your father?
Pt: I never really knew that much about my father, but as I understand it he died of a cerebral hemorrhage.
Dr: How old was he?
Pt: Oh, he must have been in his late 40s.
Dr: Was an autopsy done or anything to find out . . .
Pt: There was so little . . . there was a bad occurrence, bad divorce between our mother and father when I was real young and I never saw him after age nine months really. So I'm very hazy on the particulars of this.

The physician here stumbles on two kinds of loaded information, the one that the father died of a cerebral hemorrhage at an age that happens to be about the same age as the patient; the other that the patient does not know much because of "a bad occurrence." The physician ignores the latter and goes after his theory that the hemorrhage was caused by a berry aneurysm, of relevance to this patient because such a condition can be hereditary.

Dr: But nobody knew whether it was traumatic, did he get hit or anything?
Pt: I don't know the details, to tell you the truth. He had, well I just don't really know enough to talk about it.
Dr: Cerebral hemorrhage at a young age would be an unusual thing. No other causes being known.
Pt: I could find out more, my mother may know more about it.
Dr: If she knew, it would be important to you . . . if she would know, for instance, if he had an aneurysm in his brain that burst, which is one of the ways you can have a cerebral hemorrhage at a young age. I think that would be very important, for instance, for your general health information so perhaps you can find out. Okay? Do you know anything more in terms of other problems?

Note the physician's graphic description of "an aneurysm in his brain that burst" and the implication that this "would be very important" while quickly moving on to "other problems." The patient now goes on to talk about "the painful subject," while the physician completely ignores the affective content of the interview.

> Pt: Well, my understanding is, the context of this, that my mother was raised in the Catholic Church, and divorce was a terrible scandal in her mind and she tried to forget about it as quickly as she could. It's such a painful subject that there was never any discussion about who he was and so forth. And as a consequence, all I've really heard are niblets and one of the things I understand is that he was an alcoholic or at least had a problem with alcohol but really caused my mother a lot of problems. So, I don't know if that would be a complicating factor in terms of aneurysm or not.
>
> Dr: Not that I know of. How about brothers and sisters?
>
> Pt: I have one full natural brother and then four half brothers.
>
> Dr: Any medical problems in any of them that you know of?
>
> Pt: No.

This example, part of which was mentioned in Chapter 2, demonstrates a doctor's insensitivity to the patient's feelings and self-disclosure. It also shows that, by pursuing an item of family history, the doctor can increase his patient's anxiety and raise new questions in the patient's mind about his own health. A person who tells you that his sister had breast cancer, that his father who smoked two packs of cigarettes per day for all of his adult life developed lung cancer, or that his uncle who was an asbestos worker died from mesothelioma may feel that he also is at high risk for these diseases. The more you press for details about such illnesses in relatives, the more your patient may feel there is a connection with the illness he or she suffers at present.

You can avoid this problem by being clear about why you need the information, sensitive to the patient's responses, and informative in your explanations. **First,** you make it clear that family history is a routine part of your complete medical interview. **Second,** you listen carefully for any emotional overlay or any connections the patient may have made in his or her mind between family illnesses and the patient's own. **Third,** you demand no more detail than is required for your care of the patient. There is no point in close questioning about diseases of grandparents or in trying to determine whether a "heart attack" in an uncle was really a myocardial infarction. **Fourth,** if the patient does become anxious, you direct your attention to the anxiety. This usually means allowing the patient to express his or her concerns directly; for example, that the patient's mother died at age 42 from heart disease and now the patient herself is 41 years old and not feeling so well. Such an age coincidence is not at all uncommon, and often the patient will not have consciously made that connection. In such a case, anxiety may be "free floating" and you may need to carefully point out the coincidence of ages, while also explaining the total difference in circumstances.

Another source of anxiety rises from the psychologic bias called "availability" (see Chapter 7). An unusual illness that happens to occur in a family member is highly visible and "available" to the patient. Therefore, it has a greater impact on her fears than we might feel is justified. You look at the disease statistically and understand that it is not familial and that the chance of its occurring twice in a small number of people is extremely remote. However, you, as medical clerk, resident, or practicing physician, will find that "availability" plagues you all the time, just as it plagues your patients. After you diagnose your first case of glioblastoma multiforme, you will likely over-react to your next group of patients who complain of headaches. For the same reasons, you must be especially sensitive to the anxieties of a patient whose sister has multiple sclerosis or of the mother whose nephew had Reye's syndrome.

REVIEW OF SYSTEMS

The review of systems (ROS) demonstrates your responsibility for the total patient, and it may uncover significant problems or symptoms not otherwise elicited. It is neither a refuge nor a burden. Some physicians who feel uncertain about how to conduct an interview or about their ability to integrate data take refuge in a long, detailed ROS that uses up an inordinate amount of time and energy. They seem to be asking about every possible symptom individually and in great detail, behaving as though it were possible to get "all" the information simply by asking "all" the questions. Such a marathon is exhausting for both patients and doctors. Other physicians consider the ROS as a pro forma detail, something of little value that must be done; in other words, a burden.

It is easier to understand the ROS by first concentrating on the function it serves, rather than its content or the method of performing it. The function is simply to uncover any additional active medical problems that may or may not influence or be related to the ones for which the patient came to see the doctor. The doctor may ask questions that serve that function at any time during the interview. The ROS proper may be "emptied" when the relevant information is obtained elsewhere. Nondirective questions at the end of the "present illness" segment of the interview may obtain much of this information. For example, "Can you think of any other symptoms that you've had lately?" or "Do you have any other illnesses that have been acting up lately or are under treatment?" In this way other problems that relate to the present illness are uncovered early in the interview, thereby avoiding last-minute surprises during the 11th hour of the ROS. Another good screening question is "What medications do you take?" Whatever the patient responds to this, it is often good to ask, "Are there any other medications? How about over-the-counter or nonprescription medicines? Aspirin? Vitamins?" The past medical history sometimes also presents opportunities to explore the ROS. If the patient reports any chronic illnesses or ill-defined symptoms in the past, it is a good idea to ask if these or similar symptoms occur at present.

Platt and McMath (1979) observed more than 300 clinical interviews conducted by medical residents and delineated five syndromes of "clinical hypocompetence." One of these syndromes is called **flawed data base** and is illustrated by the following case:

> The clinical interview took 44 minutes to complete. Time allocation was as follows: introduction—1 minute; definition of chief complaint (cardinal symptom) and development of present illness—15 minutes; major past medical events, health hazards (smoking, alcohol, medications), and family illnesses—8 minutes; and review of systems—20 minutes.

In this case the interview was structured in such a way that its efficiency in generating data was very poor. A large portion of it was devoted to an ROS; this is generally unnecessary when one uses earlier parts of the interview to develop an understanding of the patient's life, habits, interests, and other active medical problems, as well as a skillful exploration of the current illness. Platt and McMath point out that a more functional allocation of time might be: introduction (1 minute); understanding the patient's life, habits, and interests (5 minutes); definition of chief complaint and present illness and (15 minutes); definition of other active medical problems (5 minutes); major past medical and family history (8 minutes); and review of systems (3 minutes). At first glance, a 3-minute ROS seems surprising if not downright impossible, but as you gain skill in asking open-ended questions early in the interview, the ROS will get shorter and shorter.

As you gain experience, much of the ROS can be conducted while you perform the physical examination. As you examine the patient's ears with your otoscope, you might ask if he or she has had any problems with hearing, ear infections, and so forth; as you examine the eyes, you might ask if he or she wears glasses. This method of doing an ROS, however, requires a high level of competence in performing the physical and the ROS so that you do not miss anything. An additional problem is that the patient may believe you are asking your question (for example, "Are you having any headaches?") based on something that you see in his eyes with your ophthalmoscope. This may create anxiety, which could change what would otherwise be neutral and accurate information. It is important to preface your examination, or at least your questions, with a statement that you will be asking routine questions for the sake of completeness rather than questions specifically related to the patient's illness or physical findings.

Many practicing physicians approach the ROS with a standardized questionnaire that the patient fills out prior to seeing the doctor. The Cornell Medical Index, for example, is one widely used questionnaire. The use of such an instrument, however, does not replace an ROS section of the interview but merely changes its character. Instead of asking about symptoms, the physician must review the questionnaire and ask for more detail about all those items for which the patient has indicated a "yes" answer. This is a perfectly acceptable format, but it is useful for the beginning physician to learn to ascertain a complete ROS without the benefit of such instruments. Then, after you have developed a comfortable style, you might create a more personalized questionnaire for future use. You must still check out **pertinent negatives**, the symptoms a patient **does not** have that would, if he or she had them, support one of your diagnostic hypotheses. You must also determine that the patient has, indeed, understood the written words well enough to answer the questions accurately.

Several guidelines are useful in learning about and conducting a good ROS. **First,** it is not necessary to ask detailed questions about every symptom related to every organ system. You can expand the net of your inquiry by first emphasizing symptoms related to the patient's principal complaints and by starting with general as opposed to yes/no questions (for example, "Are you having any trouble with your vision?" rather than "Is your vision decreasing?" or "Do you see double?"). In other words, ask the patient about general difficulty with each system, then focus in on details of existing symptoms, and finally check out pertinent negatives. **Second,** the ROS obviously should be abbreviated or eliminated in emergency situations; it can also be completed at a later date if the patient is too tired or too sick to respond to a tedious inquiry at present. **Third,** anyone, even someone in perfect health, is likely to have some positive responses on a complete ROS. In the case of each positive response, you should obtain enough detail to indicate whether positive symptoms are significant or trivial. As a general rule, significance relates to severity and duration: the more severe and the more chronic the symptom, the more likely it is to be important. **Fourth,** the use of ambiguous terms such as "indigestion," "bowel trouble," or "fatigue" is adequate for initial screening; if there are any positive responses the symptoms must then be defined more precisely. **Finally,** the separate ROS section of the history should be at the end of the interview so that you have had time earlier to "size up" the patient and ascertain how much direction the patient will need to volunteer important symptoms, whether there is denial on the one hand or obsession with the trivial on the other.

The following transcript, taken from a real patient history, provides an example of an ROS. It is neither completely comprehensive nor ideal but simply a good example conducted by a medical intern:

Dr: I'm going to ask you a bunch of questions I ask everybody. They are very general questions and some of them have short answers. Do you find that you get fevers often?

Pt: No.

Dr: How about chills? Have you had any chills recently?

Pt: Yes, but I just took that as being, you know, my hormones for my hysterectomy. That's what I took it as being.

Dr: Okay. Do you get night sweats?

Pt: Yes.

Dr: Do you soak through all your bed clothing?

Pt: No.

Dr: How much do you weigh now?

Pt: 202.

Dr: How much did you weigh a year ago?

Pt: About 180 to 190.

Dr: What is the most you have ever weighed?

Pt: This.

Dr: You certainly aren't losing weight right now. Is that right?

Pt: Right.

Dr: Do you get headaches?

Pt: Sometimes. Maybe I'd say once a month. Maybe once every other month.

Dr: Do you have problems with your vision?

Pt: No.

Dr: Do you ever see double vision?

Pt: No.

Dr: Ever see spots in front of your eyes?

Pt: No.

Dr: How about blurry vision?

Pt: No.

Dr: Have you ever passed out?

Pt: No.

Dr: Blacked out?

Pt: No.

Dr: Do you often feel light headed?

Pt: No.

Dr: Do you hear ringing in your ears?

Pt: No.

Dr: Do you get a pain in your throat?
Pt: No.
Dr: Sore throats often?
Pt: No.
Dr: Does your neck hurt?
Pt: No.
Dr: Have you noticed any lumps or bumps anywhere in your body?
Pt: No.
Dr: Do your joints ache?
Pt: Yes.
Dr: Which ones?
Pt: Here.
Dr: Okay, you are pointing to your left knee and your back. How about other joints in your body?
Pt: No.
Dr: Do your muscles ache?
Pt: I just thought that it was my muscles in my leg.
Dr: Okay, fine. Do you get short of breath when you exercise?
Pt: I haven't exercised.
Dr: How about just walking around town?
Pt: No.
Dr: Can you climb stairs without becoming short of breath?
Pt: Yes.
Dr: Do you get pain in your chest?
Pt: No.
Dr: Have you ever gotten pain in your chest while you were exercising?
Pt: No.
Dr: Have you ever felt your heart fluttering or racing very quickly?
Pt: I don't think so.
Dr: Do your ankles swell on you?
Pt: No.
Dr: Are you able to lie flat in bed without becoming short of breath?
Pt: Yes.
Dr: Do you ever wake up in the middle of the night short of breath?
Pt: No.
Dr: Do you have to cough often?
Pt: No.
Dr: Ever cough up blood?
Pt: No.
Dr: Have you noticed any change in bowel habits, your bowel functions?
Pt: Yes.
Dr: How have they changed?

Pt: I don't pass my bowels as often as I did before I had my surgery.
Dr: How often do you pass your bowels now?
Pt: Maybe twice a week.
Dr: Is the stool shaped as it was before or is it different? Is it thicker or thinner?
Pt: Thicker. Yeah because a lot of times I have to chew some Feenamints to make it go myself.
Dr: Do you have diarrhea intermixed with this at all?
Pt: No.
Dr: Have you noticed any tarry black stools?
Pt: No.
Dr: How about blood in your stools or on your stools?
Pt: No.
Dr: Have you had any belly pain?
Pt: Yeah.
Dr: Where does your belly hurt you?
Pt: Right where I had my incision. Sometimes like only when I laugh.
Dr: It hurts you along the incision?
Pt: Uh huh.
Dr: How about somewhere else in your belly?
Pt: Right here.
Dr: Okay, you are pointing to your right groin area.
Pt: It's just like —mostly like when I see something real funny and just like when I laugh. There is not any pain, it's just there. I just get a pain when I start laughing.
Dr: Have you noticed if you are very thirsty often? Do you find yourself drinking a lot of fluids?
Pt: Sometimes.
Dr: Do you think that you get cold more easily than some of your friends? Do you find that you put on clothing—heavy clothing—when other people are not wearing jackets and things?
Pt: No.
Dr: Does the heat bother you more than you think it bothers other people?
Pt: No.
Dr: What is your energy level like?
Pt: So-so. It's moderate.
Dr: Do you become fatigued easily?
Pt: Sometimes.
Dr: How's your appetite?
Pt: Great.

CHAPTER 5

The Medical History, Part 3: The Patient Profile

> Dialogue . . . can exhibit the object from each point of view, and show it to us in the round, as a sculptor shows us things, gaining in this manner all the richness and reality of effect that comes from those side issues that are suddenly suggested by the central idea in progress, and really illumine the idea more completely, or from those felicitous after-thoughts that give a fuller completeness to the central scheme, and yet convey something of the delicate charm of chance.
>
> Oscar Wilde, *The Critic as Artist. Part II*

The patient profile (also called the social history) is that part of the medical interview in which we attempt to learn something about who the patient is as a person. Illness is not simply disordered pathophysiology, when it happens to a person and involves many changes in the person's feelings and abilities. Moreover, getting sick, seeking care, getting well, and staying well all have social determinants. "Patienthood is a psychosocial, not a biologic state. A person becomes a patient by consulting a physician, or a surrogate for one, in the officially legitimated health care system" (Eisenberg, 1980). Knowledge of the patient as a person enriches the overall experience of seeing patients as well as one's understanding of the individual patient; it is essential to the biopsychosocial approach to the patient. Therapeutic decisions involve not only medical judgments but emotional, philosophic, social, and interpersonal considerations as well.

The importance of the social history may not be readily apparent in the acute hospital setting where the diagnostic and therapeutic objectives are set on an hour-to-hour (if not minute-to-minute) basis. In this artificial setting, knowing who the person is or what the illness is like for the person, seems much less important than knowing about the disease process. All this changes when it is time to discharge the patient. How many stairs will he or she have to walk up? Is the patient able to prepare or have access to the low-salt food required for his congestive heart failure? How will he or she juggle the complicated medication schedule? How much will the patient's employment allow suggested changes in lifestyle? In practice your objective is not only to get the patient out of the hospital but also to help him or her be well enough to stay out of the hospital. To do this you need to understand the impact of the disease on the person and on that person's style of living. For all stress-related illnesses, what is the impact of the patient returning to the same stressful situation that may have occasioned the hospital admission in the first place? What about diseases that are even more clearly occupational, such as back injuries in a young mother or carpal tunnel syndrome in a heavy equipment operator?

Moreover, while early in your training disease orientation tends to obscure the connection, the decision to become a patient is very much a social decision. This decision is influenced by patients' access to care, by what others in their "group" say about the symptoms, by their experiences with others who had the same symptoms (relatives, friends), and so on. Numerous investigators have documented the importance of these factors in the patient's time of request for help. Consider, for example, the "social" nature of rashes: people seek help for rashes on exposed skin earlier than for rashes obscured by clothing. School nurses send children home with "pinkeye," and this usually mild and self-limited illness shows up promptly in one's office. Some persons become patients when their symptoms become fashionable because of news stories; a recent example is premenstrual syndrome. The publicity about AIDS causes many homosexuals to seek care for mild symptoms that they would have ignored otherwise. Some patients do not seek care of their own "free will" but are forced to come by spouses or parents; these are usually difficult interactions until the patient becomes a willing participant. Adolescents and the elderly are often considered less than autonomous by parents or relatives, but they must be approached as adults in the doctor-patient relationship. In such instances, the physician must work to establish the "contract" with the patient.

We segregate the social history into its own small section of the written case history as if it were something distinct or even optional, but this is an arbitrary separation for the sake of organization only. You are continually acquiring "social" information throughout the history from "small talk," the patient's manner of dress and speech, payment method, or insurance information that may appear on the chart. In the hospital there is less access to this kind of information—there is a sameness to how people look lying in bed in hospital gowns. But what ward the patient is on, whether he or she has a private physician, normally uses clinics or emergency rooms as opposed to private practitioners, all yield clues. Another important aspect of what might be called "social history" is knowing enough about the patient to assess educational level and intelligence, both of which are critical to your ability to communicate successfully. Much of this is done automatically in the course of conversation. You want to converse at your patient's level of comprehension and not to speak in a manner inappropriate to his or her life experience.

Just as it is a mistake to believe that there is such a thing as a "complete" review of systems (there are always more questions one can ask), so it is a mistake to believe that there is a "complete" social history (there will always be more about the person that you do not know). You have time constraints. How do you limit the inquiry so as to avoid a lengthy assessment? What is relevant and what should be obtained in the limited amount of time that you have? What information must be obtained when the patient is admitted or on the first office visit, and what can wait to be developed over the course of a hospitalization or long-term relationship with the patient? You need to know at least enough to answer these three questions: (1) How does the patient's lifestyle "support" this illness? (2) How did it contribute to the illness? and (3) How will it interfere with getting well? Some illness connections with the patient's lifestyle or personality are obvious, such as the development of recurrent viral infections among daycare workers. At times, the social history is critical to making the diagnosis (AIDS is an excellent example); at other times the diagnosis is straightforward but keeping the patient well depends on his or her ability to, say, follow a special diet or complex regimen of medications.

You can begin the patient profile with questions such as: "Can you tell me a little about yourself? Your family? Your work?" or "How have things been going for you otherwise? At home? At work? In your marriage?" Try to develop a picture of the patient as a person. What is this person like? Who is he or she? What is a typical day like? Often one of the most useful parts of an entire history is a detailed description of what the patient usually does on an ordinary day and exactly how this is modified by the illness. For example, in the case of a person who may be suffering from dementia, the description of a typical day may be more revealing than all the mental status testing that one can do. It may be more important as well, as what really counts is how the patient functions in his or her environment, not on a mental status test.

A complete patient profile could be structured as given below. This is not an outline of questions to ask but a framework in which to organize information. The degree of completeness you need depends on the situation. Some of it may emerge in the course of the interview without specific questioning. Much of it is acquired not on day one of the hospitalization but over time as you get to know the patient and understand what is relevant to his or her care. Keep in mind that the idea is to find out the patient's strengths and weaknesses and the nature of his or her support system, if any. How has this person coped with illness or other stress in the past? How does he or she keep distress within manageable limits? Remember that more intimate data are more easily and reliably obtained later in the hospitalization, or years later in your relationship with the patient. Tailor what you need to know to the situation.

DEMOGRAPHICS. Patients' age, education, race or ethnic background, and residence are some of the most fundamental data about them, affecting their risk for disease as well as their beliefs about what is causing their symptoms and their ability to participate in recommended therapy.

OCCUPATION. Data about employment, school, or retirement are vital to understanding who the patient is as a person and in building an understanding of the patient's support system. For married women it is better to ask "Do you work outside your home?" than "Do you work?" Are there financial problems related to the patient's job or lack thereof? Is the retired person actively involved in hobbies or volunteer work? How does the patient cope with being a working wife and mother? How does the patient unwind from the rigors of daily living? By not considering occupational exposures, clinicians miss the opportunity to diagnose certain acute and chronic illnesses. Table 5, adapted from Goldman and Peters (1981), presents various examples of environmental causes of medical problems.

There are three essential points to a basic quick survey that can be included in any complete medical history. (1) The physician should inquire about the patient's occupation and construct a short list of jobs the patient has held, particularly those held for a long time. (2) The review of systems should include one key screening question about exposure: "Do you now (or did you sometime in the past) have exposure to fumes, chemicals, dusts, loud noise, or radiation?" (3) Some attention should be devoted to exploring any temporal relationship of the current medical problem to activities at work or at home, including job-related stress.

The key details are what the person actually does on the job. For example, a patient who "works for the phone company" may have a managerial position, may install telephones, or may do maintenance on poles outdoors. Similarly, a "steelworker" may operate heavy equipment, drive a truck, or work in a blast furnace. Each job is different and exposes the patient to different risks, ranging from chronic stress to serious accidents.

THE FAMILY. It is helpful to find out who lives at home (for example, parents, grandparents, siblings, spouse, children) and their ages. Persons who are widowed face special problems in coping with stress and, indeed, have higher rates of illness and death, particularly in the first year of widowhood. As you get to know the patient better, you can begin to discuss the stresses and satisfactions related to his or her family's functioning.

LIFESTYLE. Knowledge of the patient's demographic characteristics, occupation, and family situation will give you many clues to the patient's

TABLE 5. Examples of Environmental Causes of Medical Problems

Effects	Agent	Potential Exposures
Immediate or Short-Term:		
Dermatoses (allergic or irritant)	Metals (chromium, nickel) fibrous glass epoxy resins, cutting oils, solvents, caustic alkali, soaps	Electroplating, metal cleaning, plastic, machining, leather tanning, housekeeping
Acute psychoses	Lead (especially organic), mercury, carbon disulfide	Handling gasoline, seed handling, fungicide, wood preserving, viscose rayon industry
Asthma or dry cough	Formaldehyde, toluene diisocyanate, animal dander	Textiles, plastics, polyurethane kits, lacquer use, animal handlers
Pulmonary edema, pneumonia	Nitrogen oxides, phosgene, halogen gases, cadmium	Welding, farming ("silo filler's disease"), chemical operations, smelting
Cardiac arrhythmias	Solvents, fluorocarbons	Metal cleaning, solvent use, refrigerator maintenance
Angina	Carbon monoxide	Car repair, traffic exhaust, foundry, wood finishing
Abdominal pain	Lead	Battery making, enameling, smelting, painting, welding, ceramics, plumbing
Hepatitis (may become a long-term effect)	Halogenated hydrocarbons (e.g., carbon tetrachloride), virus	Solvent use, lacquer use, hospital workers
Latent or Long-Term:		
Chronic dyspnea Pulmonary fibrosis	Asbestos, silica, beryllium, coal, aluminum	Mining, insulation, pipefitting, sandblasting, quarrying, metal alloy work, aircraft or electrical parts
Chronic bronchitis, emphysema	Cotton dust, cadmium, coal dust, organic solvents	Textile industry, battery production, soldering, mining, solvent use
Lung cancer	Asbestos, arsenic, nickel, uranium, coke-oven emissions	Insulation, pipefitting, smelting, coke ovens, shipyard workers, nickel refining, uranium mining
Bladder cancer	β–Naphthylamine benzidine dyes	Dye industry, leather, rubber-working, chemists
Peripheral neuropathy	Lead, arsenic, β–hexane, methyl butyl ketone, acrylamide	Battery production plumbing smelting, painting, shoemaking, solvent use, insecticides
Extrapyramidal syndrome	Carbon disulfide, manganese	Viscose rayon industry, steel production, battery production, foundry
Aplastic anemia, leukemia	Benzene, ionizing radiation	Chemists, furniture refinishing, cleaning, degreasing, radiation workers

*Adapted from Goldman, R.H. and Peters, J.M.: *The occupational and environmental health history.* JAMA 246(24):2831, December 1981.

lifestyle. How the patient spends a typical day reveals even more about factors that may contribute to illness or facilitate getting well. The sedentary retired salesman will need an explicit and graded exercise program with frequent monitoring of his progress as he recuperates from a heart attack. People who are constantly on the go, eating on the run, and rarely preparing their own food may need to undertake major and difficult changes in lifestyle in order to treat their obesity and hyperlipidemia.

DIET. You may not learn much detailed, practical knowledge about nutrition during your medical education. Your patients, on the other hand, may have strong beliefs about the role of diet in their illnesses. Many will have tried specific weight reduction plans and will ask your advice about them. You will also be recommending changes, such as salt restriction or reduction in saturated fats, for treatment of your patients with chronic diseases. If you have no idea about the person's basic eating habits, you will be making these recommendations in an abstract way, rather than being able to give specific advice about certain foods. All this means that the nutritional part of your patient profile can be important and sometimes, in health maintenance and prevention, it can yield your most effective interventions for the patient.

You should find out how many meals per day the person usually eats and roughly at what times. You should also learn what sort of snacks your patient eats on a daily basis. You will encounter obese patients who tell you, quite sincerely, that they eat only one meal per day. They attempt to cut down and lose weight but are continually frustrated in their efforts. "I hardly eat anything, yet everything I eat turns to fat . . . I just can't lose a pound." Part of this problem arises from their one-meal-per-day habit, which promotes frequent (sometimes continual) snacking during other times of the day. This snacking may be an almost unconscious background phenomenon that the person really fails to consider. Another factor contributing to this failure to lose weight is that very obese people tend to be quite sedentary in their lifestyles. They may need relatively few calories and so will find it truly difficult to "cut down" to a level of intake below the calories they are burning up daily.

Another aspect of dietary history is a general picture of its composition. You should find out roughly (a) the proportion of red meat in the diet, as compared to poultry or fish; (b) other saturated fats in the diet (butter or margarine, dairy products, cooking oils); (c) some indication of indigestible fiber intake (grains, leafy vegetables); and (d) preferences for salt cooked in food and/or added to food. Special consideration should also be given to caffeine in the diet. Our society is hooked on coffee and caffeine-containing soft drinks. It is not uncommon to find patients who drink several cups of coffee per day routinely, in addition to frequent cola beverages, and who increase this intake during periods of stress. Caffeine usage may be a crucial factor for patients who come in with upper gastrointestinal symptoms, headaches, irritability, fatigue, and lightheadedness.

SUPPORT SYSTEM. With the answers to the previous questions you are beginning to develop an idea of the patient's support system. Are there family members nearby who are willing and able to help in time of crisis? What kind of help does the young mother have with her new baby? Who will care for the elderly demented lady when her husband (who normally cares for her) has his hernia surgery? Most chronic illnesses, any illness that results in disability, as well as psychiatric disorders, require the physician to know who is available to help the patient get well and stay well. When there is no family or the family has limited financial or emotional resources, it is necessary to involve social agencies to provide services ranging from transportation to doctor's appointments to meals in the home.

IMPACT OF ILLNESS. Illness may affect the patient in many ways—both trivial and profound. There are the day-to-day problems, such as getting up and down steps for a patient whose surgery or illness limits her ability to do so in a house with its only bathroom on the second floor; or the widower who eats out and must limit his sodium intake. Illness produces hardships of a different sort when it takes away the patient's ability to earn a living or renders the aging spouse unable to care for her mate. Illnesses also have an emotional impact; a woman with a localized breast cancer and a man with an uncomplicated acute myocardial infarction may well have the same good prognosis, but in our society a diagnosis of cancer is usually more devastating than a diagnosis of heart disease. For some, illness has positive consequences, such as for the person who believes physical suffering leads to spiritual enlightenment. For others, illness may represent a concrete sign of their failure to pray correctly or to have sufficient faith in God to be "healed."

MARITAL AND/OR SIGNIFICANT RELATIONSHIPS. As you begin to understand the patient's lifestyle and the impact of the illness, you will also be developing a sense of the patient's relationship with his or her spouse or "significant other." You may not need to ask direct questions about this. Because patients may regard this sort of information as intimate and possibly unrelated to their illness, it is best to ask questions in a somewhat indirect and open-ended manner, which permits patients to answer in their own terms, revealing as much or as little as they wish. Start with questions that relate the patient's illness to the current state of the relationship, such as "How has your doing home dialysis affected your husband?" Then proceed to more intimate questions, such as "How have 20 years of married life been?" Such questions allow the patient to say anything from "Okay" to "Well, we've had our rough spots but things are pretty good right now" to "To tell you the truth, I keep wanting to leave him but I can't." Still more specific questions, such as "What are some of the good and bad things about your present relationship?" or "What would you change?" are useful once the patient has indicated an interest in discussing the relationship. Sexual behavior and illness influence each other in many ways and may have an impact on significant relationships. We consider the sexual history in detail in Chapter 8.

CIGARETTE, ALCOHOL, AND ILLICIT DRUG USE. These "social" habits are often listed as part of the social history. While these data may be obtained in that part of the interview, smoking and casual use of alcohol more properly belong in the medications or review of systems part of the interview. Illicit drug use and alcohol abuse are illnesses in their own right and are also "social" problems for the patient, the family, and society at large. One should ascertain the amount, frequency, situations of use, and reasons for use. We consider the drug and alcohol history in detail in Chapter 8.

Next we consider some examples that demonstrate the importance of the social history or patient profile in the diagnosis and management of medical problems. In this first example, a 61-year-old black woman with known diabetes and hypertension urgently scheduled a visit to her family physician, complaining of chest pain, headache, and increasing concern about her blood pressure. The physician, confused about which problem was really the chief complaint, since the symptoms were chronic and the blood pressure well controlled, asked the patient to clarify her concerns:

Dr: Uh, what, what would you say is the thing that's worrying you the most right now?
Pt: Well, mostly, is how, getting those bills paid. See, I'm on, I'm on assistance.
Dr: Oh, I see. Tell me more about this worry. Did something new happen?
Pt: Mostly it's a gas bill and then, um, see I own a house. I have the taxes, keeping up with them, and, ah, just finances generally.
Dr: Did you recently get your gas bill?
Pt: Yes I did.
Dr: When did that come?
Pt: Yes, ah, it came the other day.

In this instance, the "social" problem was the problem. Notice how the physician went after positive or confirmatory evidence that there were, indeed, data to support the notion that it was her inability to pay the gas bill that was really bothering the patient. This does not mean that the patient did not have "real" chest pain, headaches, and high blood pressure; but it was very helpful in answering the "why now" question, why the patient sought care **now** for symptoms that had not changed.

Next, consider this example, in which another kind of social determinant of the decision to seek care becomes apparent:

> Pt: See, um, I used to, okay, I used to do hair, I'm a barber, I'd do a lotta hair, so I had to go to, uh, um, I had to go to the clinic. Okay, now barbers every time they get their license renewed, they have to go to the health department.
> Dr: Right.
> Pt: Right. Okay and they gave, uh, they gave me some pills to take because they gave me a test, um, humm, and it came back positive . . .
> Dr: Um humm.
> Pt: You know they gave me some pills to take, they say I have to take them for a year.
> Dr: Um humm.
> Pt: But before the end of the year, after I run out, I'm supposed to come back and get some more . . .
> Dr: Right, I see . . .
> Pt: And I didn't.

Here, the patient who has chest pain is probably concerned that his failure to follow up on recommended treatment for what was a positive tuberculin test may be the etiology of his current symptoms. The only reason he had the tuberculin test in the first place was to satisfy the state licensing requirements to be a barber.

Here is another example, in which the patient describes a bout of gastrointestinal symptoms:

> Dr: Do you think that a week ago when you had this vomiting that you had some kind of virus or flu bug?
> Pt: I could of had a little bit of a slight—I ate some food that wasn't real fresh and it could of been that, plus maybe—I don't know what it was. It could of been the food I ate.
> Dr: How was it that you ate some food that wasn't so fresh?
> Pt: Well, my refrigerator is bad and it's been so hot, I don't have the money to fix it.

The physician is rightly concerned about how it was that the patient came in contact with possibly offensive food; a bad refrigerator is a "social" problem that can lead to disease. Let us close with an example of a patient who has numerous influences on his life that are contributing to his illnesses, which include obesity, headaches, and secondary syphilis:

Pt: The thing that is interesting to me is I am busy and I am constantly on my feet and I must put in at least 4 miles each day, but it doesn't affect my weight because of the types of things I eat. I don't eat heavily, it's just the things I eat.

Dr: How do you mean?

Pt: When I have not eaten for a whole day I go to some deli and grab a cream puff and go to bed. That gives me sugar and sugar helps me. Sugar really helps me keep elevated. I have a terrible—well, I have to drink orange drink. I don't eat breakfast, as a matter of fact, I only eat one meal a day, but it's a junk meal. And I'm very hooked on, I have to have a sugar-type drink in the morning to get elevated. Could use one now!

Dr: Now that you know all these things, is there any way you can change something? Like when you go to New York, you can find some time for yourself, even if it's sitting down for 10 minutes instead of 10 seconds?

Pt: I lived there for two years and when I started the business, I didn't realize at the time that the business was going to grow as quickly as it did and I found out I was going to New York more and staying in hotels. Hotel living is disgusting. All I want to do is—my day starts at usually six-thirty or seven o'clock in the morning and sometimes ends at ten or eleven at night. And all I want to do is go back to the hotel, shove some sugar in my face, and go to sleep. This is the part where it gets into the personal part of it. My lifestyle changed quite a bit; a lot of things changed for me. I have always felt that I had very strong religious convictions and things like that. When I moved to New York, my lifestyle totally changed. I had to be very social; I wasn't a drug person. But I went to parties where everybody was having sex with everybody else and you really didn't even get to know the person. You may never see them again and that type of thing. Well, all these things happened to me in this period. And I have to be honest with you, they frightened me but I enjoyed them. I knew they were wrong, but there was a part of me that enjoyed them. So I was getting very confused. I felt that it was time for me to come back.

Dr: You felt that this was a way of coming back home?

Pt: Exactly. What happened to me recently was that because of me going back to the way I wanted to be and things not working out the way I thought they should, so I figured why should I make sacrifices and be this person? You know, and not getting the results I want from it. I'll go back to being the other person. And I went back to being the other person and I got (laughing loudly) a social disease! Now you know my life story. That's it in a nutshell.

This patient had numerous social influences contributing to his diseases. He probably acquired syphilis at a party at which he had multiple sexual partners; he was finding his obesity difficult to control and was experiencing constant fatigue and stress-related tension (muscle contraction) headaches. His syphilis, which had advanced to the secondary stage with the development of a rash before it was diagnosed, required hospitalization and became very public evidence of what the patient saw as transgressions. When the news about AIDS hit, he became dreadfully afraid that he had been exposed to the AIDS virus because of his contacts with homosexuals who had numerous sexual partners. His anxiety about contracting a lethal disease (and his guilt) made it very difficult for him to work as hard as he felt he needed to in order to keep his business going.

CHAPTER 6

The Transition to the Physical Examination and Closure

> . . . A physician of this kind never gives a servant any account of his complaint, nor asks him for any; he gives him some empirical injunction with an air of finished knowledge in the brusque fashion of a dictator, and then is off in hot haste to the next ailing servant . . .
>
> Plato, *The Laws*

Medical interviewing, unlike other forms of the helper-client interaction, usually also involves a physical examination. The history and physical examination are different parts of the same process, a process that also includes negotiation, education, and clarification of plans. If we focus on data gathering, it is difficult to pinpoint exactly when the history ends and the physical examination begins, or vice versa. For example, from the first moment the patient walks into your office or you walk into the patient's hospital room, you begin to make observations about the physical condition of the patient: you observe skin color, affect, behavior, and mental status. The entire "mental status examination," although part of the interview in that it involves no touching, is really more properly considered as part of the systematic "physical examination." On the other side of the coin, as you are doing the physical examination you continue to interact with your patient, hoping to obtain not only "physical" but also personal information.

TRANSITION TO THE PHYSICAL EXAMINATION

It is difficult at first to go from talking to touching. Early in your medical experience it is especially difficult to unglue yourself from your chair and approach the patient. You can handle this transition with a statement like "I'd like to examine you now—if you're not too tired." In the hospital other attention to the patient's comfort, such as offering some water or changing the window blinds, may be appropriate.

Ordinarily, when in the clinic or in your office, you will be interviewing a patient who is fully clothed. Although having a patient disrobe and put on an examination gown prior to the medical history is often conducive to good office functioning, it is rarely conducive to patient comfort. It undermines respect for the person. Thus, the patient should be fully clothed and you will be faced with telling him or her to get undressed when you are ready to start the examination. You should be quite direct and clear about what is going to happen and why. **First,** give the patient an opportunity for the last word: "I think that's about it for now. Is there anything else we haven't covered or that you'd like to tell me before I examine you?" **Second,** tell the patient clearly what the game plan is: "Next, I'm going to do your physical examination, and then after that we can sit down and talk about your problems and what tests you might need." **Third,** be very specific about what clothing the patient should remove, where he or she should sit or lie, and in what position. For example, "I'm going to step out of the room for a moment now. Please get undressed down to your underpants and put on this gown. Put it on with the opening toward the back. And then sit on the end of the table up here." Here is how one physician begins an examination of a woman she is seeing for the first time. Note the explicit directions as well as a "review of systems" type question as she begins the examination:

> Dr: Do you have any questions before we do your exam?
> Pt: No.
> Dr: Okay. Why don't you climb up here, and just sit there, just step around, and come around there. Okay. I am going to cover you and you can just sit there first. I am going to check your thyroid and your lungs and your heart, and examine your breasts. Have you had any thyroid trouble?
> Pt: No.

It is best for you to leave the room, or to pull a curtain across the room if one is available, while your patient gets undressed. In the hospital, of course, this is usually not a problem but, even there, patients may want to use the bathroom and/or remove a dressing gown or robe. In office practice, when you are only doing part of a physical examination, it may be appropriate for the patient to remove only his or her shirt or to unbutton several buttons. For specific parts of the examination, ask the patient to disrobe that area or, alternatively, say, "I'm going to untie (unbutton, remove) . . ." If a female patient has large breasts, ask her for assistance in moving the breast in order for you to listen to the heart. This helps the patient to feel more like a participant and less like a victim.

CONVERSATION DURING THE PHYSICAL EXAMINATION

While conversation during the physical examination allows you to continue to gather data, it may serve other essential functions as well. You can use your communication skills to put the patient at ease, encourage the patient to feel like an active participant in his or her own care, and diminish the power differential between physician and patient, which becomes more marked during the physical examination. Here is how one patient described it:

> Whether it be horizontal, or in some awkward placement on one's back or stomach, with legs splayed or cramped, or even in front of a desk, the patient is placed in a series of passive, dependent, and often humiliating positions. These are positions where embarrassment and anger are at war with the desire to take in what the doctor is saying. In this battle learning is clearly the loser. (Eisenberg and Kleinman, 1980)

You can also use conversation to show the patient that you remember his complaint about abdominal pain while you are doing the abdominal exam; or you may use "small talk" to distract the patient so her muscles will relax, making the abdominal or pelvic exam easier for her and more accurate as well.

Keep talking during the examination to gather further information, to reassure the patient, and to explain what you are doing. It may not be possible as a beginner to make comments while you are also concentrating on the sequence of things to do and the techniques for doing them. It is not difficult, however, to make such observations as:

> "I'm going to look into your ears now."

> "I'm feeling for your thyroid gland. Can you swallow now? I know it's difficult to swallow like that when someone asks you. Good."

> "I'm going to do a rectal exam now to check your prostate gland. It will make you feel like you are going to have a bowel movement— but don't worry, you won't."

It is also not very difficult for you, while being very reassuring for the patient, to indicate that parts of your examination are normal. It is usually not particularly helpful to comment on every little thing you do, but if you know the patient is concerned about a particular system, it would be helpful to note your findings about that system right away. For the patient who comes in with chest pain, a comment that the heart and lungs sound normal can be quite reassuring for the patient (who need not be bothered at this point with the academic information that the heart may sound normal even when there is heart disease, such as angina pectoris). Here is an example of how a physician speaks to a patient during the parts of the physical examination that involve listening to the lungs and heart, and palpating the breasts and abdomen. Notice the intervening of a few ROS-type questions as the physician examines that part, education about self breast exam, and attention to the patient's comfort ("Tell me if I hit any sore places"):

Dr: Okay, I am just going to loosen this *(unties gown in back)*. How long have you been smoking?

Pt: About three years . . .

Dr: And you want to quit.

Pt: Well, yeah, I been thinking about it.

Dr: Take a deep breath. Okay, out, good, and again . . . Good. Now I am going to ask you to slip your arms all the way out and I am going to listen to your heart . . . Okay. Sounds good. Now I'm going to check your breasts. I want you to put your hands up like this *(doctor demonstrates)* and I'm just going to look at them first to see if there are any bumps . . .

Pt: Uh mm.

Dr: Okay, have you ever tried it?

Pt: No, not really.

Dr: We recommend that everyone do it once a month, the best time is right after your period has stopped. Do your breasts get sore before your period?

Pt: Yes.

Dr: Okay, well some women do and that is why it is best to wait until after your period starts when usually the lumpiness goes away and they're not tender to touch . . . I am going to ask you to just hold this up . . . and I want you to put your arms up over your head. What you do when you are checking is to do exactly what I'm doing . . . Go all around the outside of your breasts like this . . . up here is breast tissue and also up here . . . so you are going to go in kind of a circle like this . . . then spiral in until you get every part including under the nipple. Okay? Now I'd like you to lie down and we'll check your breast again . . . we always check them in two positions . . . And I am going to check your heart . . . Do you have any indigestion or trouble with your bowels? Now tell me if I hit any sore places.

The pelvic examination is a particularly personal and anxiety-producing experience. You should explain clearly what you are about to do and what the patient is likely to feel. Ask the patient if she has had a pelvic examination before. Whether she has or not, it is very reassuring to say something like "I'm going to pretend that this is your first pelvic and explain everything that I'm doing." The less experience the patient has had either with pelvic exams or with you, the more reassurance she will need. You should first touch the patient's inner thigh and then firmly but gently conduct the examination. You should describe the anatomy to the patient as you are doing the examination. As you become more experienced, you will be able to help her relax her muscles through your calm tone of voice, your gentle palpation, and your instructions about deep, slow breathing.

Here is how one physician introduces a patient (who requests a diaphragm for birth control) to her first pelvic exam; everything is described with a relaxing, almost hypnotic, tone of voice, the physician's gestures are slow and deliberate (no sudden moves), and she continuously looks at the patient's face to gauge her reactions:

Dr: The next thing I am going to do is a pelvic exam. These are all the things I am going to use but I am not going to use all of them on you. Okay. These are the slides on which the Pap test is done, and these are the swabs that I use to do the Pap test—they're just like long Q-tips, okay, and this also which I will roll around the cervix, just like that *(demonstrating)*, see it is not sharp . . . We usually do a culture for infection at the same time . . .

Pt: A culture?

Dr: Yes, and that is to check for infection. This instrument is cold and that is really the worst thing about it. It is called a speculum and this is inserted very gently into the vagina and then opened very gently like that *(demonstrating)* so that I can see your cervix and see that it is normal. Okay?

(Patient nods.)

Dr: What I will ask you to do is to put your feet into these things which are called stirrups, these metal things, that is good, and now I want you to pull yourself all the way down to the end of the table like that, and practically feel yourself like your bottom is coming off the end of the table. Okay? That's fine. I am going to put this pillow under your head right there, okay, and I am going to shine a light on you so that I can see what I am doing and as I do things I will tell you what I am doing. Okay? Are you more or less comfortable?

Pt: I guess so.

Dr: All right, it is not very comfortable, that is true. Okay. Now what I am going to do is to look at the outside of you first. If you can just kind of relax, that's good. Now what I am doing is checking the labia, or lips. Good. Now you are going to feel my finger at the edge of the vagina, feeling where your cervix is. Do you know what your cervix is?

Pt: No.

Dr: Okay, that is the opening to your womb or uterus. Okay, I am just kind of locating it first, and that is just my finger again. Okay, now you're going to feel the cold metal which I tried to warm up a little bit, but usually it's still cold. Is that okay?

Pt: Mm hmm.

Dr: Now I insert it just until I can see your cervix so that I can do the Pap test. Okay, now I can see your cervix very clearly now and . . .

Pt: Is that where I put the diaphragm?

Dr: Exactly, that is exactly where to put the diaphragm. Okay, now I am just using one of those long Q-tips to do the Pap test, okay?

Pt: Mm hmm.

Dr: And now I'm going to use one of those scrapes and sometimes you feel that scraping feeling, but usually what you feel is the pressure of the speculum being in place there . . . Now I am just spraying those glass slides that I just took and that preserves them so they can be checked later. And now I am taking the speculum out. Are you still with me?

Pt: Yeah.

Dr: Okay, the next thing I am going to do is check your rectum and that will make you feel as though you have to have a bowel movement, right, that is just my finger in your rectum. That's kind of an uncomfortable feeling with some people. It feels completely normal. Now I am going to just check back inside your vagina, okay, and where my fingers are is where you put the diaphragm. Now I am going to ask you that when you go home you practice feeling where your cervix is. I am touching it right now. On you, it is a little bit off to your left side, okay, and it feels like the tip of your nose when you touch it. Okay. When I put one hand over here and between the two hands I can feel where your uterus is . . . And I am touching it right now and it feels normal. Now I am checking on each side for your ovaries . . .

Pt: Can you feel all that?

Dr: You can feel all that, especially in someone like you, because you are very relaxed and I can feel everything.

Notice how the physician keeps talking but frequently checks back with the patient and is educating the patient all the while about her body and about the normality of the findings. Indeed, the proof that the technique is effective is in the patient's pleasure and wonderment ("Can you feel all that?") at the ability of a pelvic examination to tell a physician so much and at her ability to completely relax her muscles.

Your continued "interview" with the patient provides clarification and reassurance. The new information aspect will gradually develop as you become more comfortable with the procedures of physical examination, so that concentration on the actual techniques can sink into the background and you are able to concentrate more thoroughly on your immediate observations. Until you are experienced, do not try to do the complete ROS during the physical examination. But if you are looking at the eyes, for example, and this reminds you of an eye question you forgot to ask, go ahead and ask it. The physical examination is also a good time to find out more about the person's life and lifestyle. Such "small talk" yields pertinent information as well as making the patient more relaxed by distracting him or her.

USES OF THE PHYSICAL EXAMINATION

What are the purposes of the physical examination? What diagnostic or therapeutic value does it serve? **First,** of course, the physical examination allows us to obtain more data to complement and supplement the history. It yields a different kind of data, **signs** rather than **symptoms.** The signs serve to confirm the hypotheses that we are beginning to develop from the history, or to dis-confirm them, or perhaps to suggest entirely different hypotheses. The physical examination, in this sense, should be as flexible and targeted as the history. In the physical examination, as in the ROS, we should not obsessively attempt to make all possible observations but only those that are relevant to the problems at hand.

Table 6 lists frequently observed errors in physical examination, based on a study of medical house officers (Weiner and Nathanson, 1976). Some are errors in technique, simply not performing the procedure correctly; some are procedures omitted inappropriately; some are errors in classification or detection, missing a sign that is really present or asserting that a sign is present when it really is not; and some are problems in interpretation, recognizing the sign but failing to recognize its value or meaning. These will be useful to review. It is comforting to know that other medical students and young physicians have the same problems with physical examination as you do. Physical examination courses have, in the past, emphasized students "doing it" on their own, usually examining hospitalized patients, and then reporting findings to their preceptors. The preceptor had little opportunity to observe the student and to teach correct techniques in this process. Skillful physical diagnosis requires not just experience (it is easy to perform the same egregious errors habitually!) but also guided instruction. Request that your preceptor observe your examinations periodically, even if you do not think you need it.

TABLE 6. Errors Most Frequently Made in Physical Examination

Type of Error	Head and Neck Examination	Chest Examination	Abdominal, Genital, and Extremity Examination	Neurologic Examination
Technique	Bimanual palpation of head and neck Determination of tracheal position Measurement of jugular venous pressure Hepatojugular reflux venous pulse waves	Palpation of expansion Percussion of diaphragm movements Auscultation for low sounds and murmurs	Palpation of spleen Deep abdominal structures Popliteal pulses Testes Percussion of liver and spleen and auscultation for bruits	Visual fields Calorics Corneal reflexes Tendon reflexes and Babinski testing
Omission	Auscultation of neck vessels Inspection of retina, cornea, lens, iris Inspection of nasal cavity	Auscultation of lateral chest and apices Cardiac auscultation in various positions Use of Valsalva and respiratory maneuvers Following radiation of murmurs	Palpation of spleen in right lateral decubitus Palpation of prostate, ovaries, kidneys Measurement of liver size by percussion Pelvic and rectal examination	Testing olfaction Hearing Corneal reflex Sensation Calorics
Detection	Thyroid nodules Tracheal deviation Bruits Oral ulcers Scleral icterus Breath odors	Decreased expansion of chest Palpation of crepitus from rib fracture Decreased breath sounds Bronchial breathing Cardiac dullness Mitral diastolic murmurs, grade 1 aortic diastolic murmurs, S_3, S_4, grade 1 systolic murmurs Fine rales	Minimal splenomegaly Palpation of enlarged kidney, gallbladder, and accurate identification Small hernias and prostatic nodules Aortic aneurysms 3- to 5-cm masses	Organic mental syndromes Aphasias Mild paresis Conjugate and disconjugate occular defects
Interpretation	Tracheal deviation Jugular pressure Skin turgor Venous pulses	Bronchial breathing Systolic murmurs Use of ancillary signs such as fremitus or whispered voice	Abdominal tenderness Transmitted pulsation vs aneurysm in the epigastrium Masses, intra-abdominal wall vs abdominal wall Venous flow patterns Liver size	Eye signs Patterns of sensory loss or weakness Reflex differences between sides

Second, the physical examination also serves as a screening device through which we can obtain information about asymptomatic disease, or about problems not mentioned by the patient during the interview. In this sense it is somewhat like a physical version of the ROS. Only a few parts of the physical examination serve in a purely screening function; that is, permit the detection of completely asymptomatic disease. In adults, these are (1) taking the blood pressure, (2) breast examination in women, (3) examination of the skin for suspicious lesions, (4) Pap smear for cervical cytology in women, and (5) rectal examination with a test for occult blood in the stool.

The physical examination, as we have indicated earlier, also provides an opportunity to continue the interview under new circumstances. It allows us to ask specifically about things we observe and thus generate new information. Our examination of a certain part of the body, perhaps the ears, may stimulate the patient to remember ear pain or ear infection he or she had not discussed when asked about past illness; likewise, we have an opportunity to ask about old surgical or traumatic scars. Musculoskeletal examination of persons who have joint or muscle complaints will allow us to inquire further about specific limitations caused by pain or weakness.

Finally, physical examination itself has a therapeutic role. Simply touching the patient—the "laying on of hands"—may cause him or her to feel better and to be reassured. Tactile communication opens up a channel of interpersonal response that can be very important in healing. In particular, specific attention to the painful areas of the body demonstrates that you have listened, understood, and are concerned about the patient's suffering.

Your systematic touching of the patient, however, does present certain risks. Such contact is a violation of taboos in our society, outside the realm of intimacy. You have a privileged role that is charged with meaning for the patient. The patient is ill and vulnerable; you are powerful. In a sense, the patient sees you as holding the keys to health or illness. You may be viewed as the messenger who can carry bad news or good news, the seer who can understand secrets of the body, or the conduit of power over illness. This charged relationship leads to several risks in doing the physical examination:

1. Inadequate preparation without appropriate attention to the patient's comfort and modesty may result in feelings of exposure or violation for the patient.
2. Appearing to neglect the patient's major concern while exploring physical findings in another area (such as examining the ear of a patient who comes in with a stomach complaint) may lead to feelings of being ignored or misunderstood.
3. Instilling fear or anxiety when a certain area of the physical exam-

ination is emphasized (such as prolonged listening to the heart) may lead the patient to believe something may be drastically wrong.

All of these dangers can be minimized by adequate preparation and explanation to the patient.

TOUCHING

We referred earlier to the fact that performing a physical examination actually has therapeutic value in itself. Patients very commonly will not be quite satisfied until you have examined them—perhaps only taking their blood pressure and listening to their heart—even when they return to your office for a follow-up visit during which no examination is medically necessary. We believe there are two components to the therapeutic value of examination, one arising from cultural expectations about what a doctor in our society does, and the other arising from the more elemental fact of touching itself.

You often have patients who say, "My stomach has felt terrible for weeks, but this morning, just as I was coming in to see the doctor, it's not hurting anymore . . ." This phenomenon of the tooth feeling better on the expectation of seeing a dentist, or the pain disappearing just prior to a visit with the doctor, is part of the symbolic healing dimension (see Chapter 11) that permeates all patient care situations. Another aspect of it is the therapeutic value of diagnostic tests. Some patients will find that their back pain improves after being assured that their lumbosacral spine x-ray results are normal. Other, less-educated patients sometimes overtly confuse diagnostic studies with therapeutic procedures: "I've felt good ever since I had that x-ray."

Everyone knows that doctors do physical examinations and can "read" the clues they find in so doing. Physical examination is part of the **therapeutic context** of medicine in our culture. Therefore, it can have a strong symbolic effect that may contribute to healing, but that may also cause iatrogenic ("from the doctor") suffering. For example, the doctor who lingers a long while over cardiac auscultation and finally announces gravely that the patient has a heart murmur, and then tells the patient he had better see a cardiologist, has really caused some anxiety which need not have existed. This may in some cases be inevitable, but it can always be minimized by full explanation to the patient in the context of empathic communication. Other aspects of the therapeutic context, including physical examination, will be discussed in Chapter 11 dealing with placebo effects.

The "laying-on-of-hands" has always been an important component of healing. Healing by touch was once thought to be a divine attribute of kings. Most traditional forms of medicine involve some component of touch in their armamentarium. The contemporary holistic health movement has spawned many forms of therapy that rely on touch, methods ranging from reflexology to the school of "therapeutic touch." Some observers believe that a major factor in chiropractic's appeal and its success has to do with the physical contact involved in chiropractic examination and spinal adjustment (Coulehan, 1985).

We cannot speculate here on the full meaning of touch, but it clearly can have great psychologic benefit if used appropriately. Whether, or by what means, this translates into physiologic benefit is unknown. Certainly, we cannot equate all touch: a cursory auscultation of the heart is far different from a detailed, careful musculoskeletal examination. Touch that arises because you and the patient are "connecting" and you feel you need to reach out (as when you put your hand over the hand of a crying patient) may well have far different therapeutic value than the touch involved in routine diagnostic procedures.

Our chief goal here is to emphasize the potential value of touch and to point out that, in general, you should not shy away from physical contact with your patient. You should use it for its symbolic value, even when you believe it will have no diagnostic value. The physician who pays special attention to touching each patient as he makes hospital rounds will likely find that this brief physical contact will help establish better understanding and more empathic communication in their relationship. This can involve something as simple as putting a hand on the patient's shoulder as you speak with him or her, listening to the patient's heart beat even though the monitor is on and there is almost no "practical" reason for doing so, or stopping for a moment and placing your hand on the patient's hand as you make a routine inquiry. Doctors who do this will find that their patients perceive that their physician spends considerably more time with them and explains things much better, even though they spend exactly the same amount of **clock time** and explain things in exactly the same way as other physicians who never make an effort to touch their patients unless necessary for a diagnostic procedure.

ENDING THE INTERVIEW

This section could be subtitled "How to Get Out of the Room Without Leaving a Lot of Loose Ends and With a Good Feeling on Your Part and That of the Patient." You have completed the physical examination and now, in a sense, "reconvene" the interview in order to terminate it. The goal of a good closure is no different from the goal of your entire interview and will be easier to attain if the patient understands from the outset the purpose of the interaction and who you are. The purpose of the interaction will vary, depending on whether you are a student in a physical diagnosis course with a one-time "shot" at the patient, a clinical clerk with major responsibility for communicating with the patient, or the resident or attending physician with a long-term role in the patient's management. Overall, the patient (and you) should expect nothing more than to feel understood and not be abused in any way. In history taking this means (1) that you have gotten the story straight, and (2) that the patient has not been forced to expose himself or herself either personally or physically without your appropriate concern for his or her comfort and modesty. The techniques of being accurate, empathic, respectful, and genuine apply to this part of the encounter as they do to all the others.

It is always a good idea to give the patient the opportunity to have the last word:

"Anything else?"

"Do you feel there is anything about what you have told me that I have not understood?"

"Is there anything else you'd like to tell me or ask me?"

As in all other aspects of clinical examination, what you do to close the encounter depends on (1) who you are—your status, how much responsibility you have in the care of the patient, as well as your own style; (2) who the patient is—his or her expectations and needs (emotional, physical); (3) what the illness is—simple versus complicated, mild versus severe, benign versus malignant, acute versus chronic, curable versus terminal.

In your role as a student learning about medical interviewing or taking a physical diagnosis course, when you close any encounter with a patient you should:

1. Provide a summary of what the patient has told you.
2. Be sure to let the patient have the last word, or ask any additional questions.
3. Give a pleasant thank you and goodbye.

This is fine with most patients, especially if you have been careful all along to clarify your role. If a patient asks a question you cannot answer about the disease or about his or her medical care, you should say something like "I am not able to answer that, but it is a good question to ask your doctor." This is a truthful answer whether the reason that you are unable to answer is that you do not know or that you do know but the question is more properly answered by the patient's physician.

Once you have responsibility for patient care, the more typical closure implies a contract between you and the patient. It acknowledges responsibility for solving problems and providing care. In this general context, ending a patient encounter, whether it be a complete history and physical or a short office visit, should include these actions on the part of the physician:

1. **Share findings.** By this we usually mean the physical findings and your diagnosis, differential diagnosis, or hypotheses. As a student you are unable to share much, as you are often unsure about your findings or diagnosis; when you become a physician the question is always **what** to share. What you share depends on the one hand on the patient: how sick he or she is, how knowledgeable, whether or not he or she has other sources of information. What you share also depends on the illness; some findings are pertinent to the illness, while others are incidental or may be trivial. Avoid discussing what is interesting to you but may be irrelevant to the patient.

2. **Devise a problem list with priorities.** This is painstaking and difficult at first but becomes easier with experience. How you do it is not the subject of this book, but it is important to realize that the doctor's priorities often differ from those of the patient. Patients may be interested first in feeling better, second in their overall prognosis, and third in the specific diagnosis. Doctors do share these same concerns but often (especially while in medical school or in training) are more interested in making the diagnosis than in treating the symptoms. Treating the symptom is often not the same as treating the disease. Many trivial illnesses do not in themselves need specific medications but have symptoms that patients want treated. On the other hand, many significant illnesses have no symptoms but demand (from the doctor's point of view) specific therapy.

3. **Agree on a plan of action and clarify responsibilities.** Determine what will happen next and who will do what. The physician may agree to order and interpret tests, talk with consultants, write prescriptions, do procedures or further history and physical. The patient may agree to take the prescription, modify diet, keep the following appointment, report further symptoms. Responsibilities are often blurred, especially in the patient who says, "I'm in your hands, Doc." Ideally, medical care is a partnership in which you negotiate an agreement or contract with the patient, but the character of that contract depends on the patient's illness (emergency care versus chronic antihypertensive therapy) and on the patient's acceptance of responsibility (see the discussion about negotiation, Chapter 10).

4. **Educate the patient.** The physician should tell the patient as much as he or she knows about the problem, within the limits of what the patient wants to know and can accept and understand. This is easier to say than to do and is not a one-shot thing but a process over time, as the physician learns about the patient and his or her problems. It is different for each physician, each patient, and each illness.

To conclude this chapter, here is an example of the closing minutes of an office visit (the patient suffers from back pain):

Dr: I don't find anything, on my exam. I don't find anything that makes me think you have a pinched nerve. I think periodically you may be getting some nerve irritation and that's accounting for the pain that's shooting down your legs. What I think we should do, I want to check your x-rays that you had. I want to review those. I think we're going to have to get you at bed rest for a while and just get you off of your feet. At least for a short time. Maybe three, four, or five days. Is that, are you able to do that?

Pt: Yeah.

Dr: You don't live by yourself?

Pt: No. I live with my daughter.

Dr: Okay, fine. I'm going to give you a couple of different medicines. I'll refill the Darvocets, but I only want you to use that as needed. I'm going to give you another medicine called Motrin. Are you able to take aspirin?

Pt: Yes.

Dr: So, I'm going to give you Motrin which is an anti-inflammatory medicine. I don't want you to expect any overnight relief from the Motrin because it takes several days, sometimes up to a week. So I'm going to give you the Motrin, Darvocet, and I'll give you a prescription for something called Pericolace, which is a very mild laxative and stool softener to make sure while you're . . . while you're down in bed rest that you don't get constipated. Do you have a heating pad at home?

Pt: Yeah, I have a moist heating pad.

Dr: Wonderful. You can use that every hour if you like, but I don't want you using it for more than 20 minutes at a time. But you can use it up to 20 minutes out of every hour. All right? So, I want you at bed rest, well I actually would like you at bed rest for a week. I want to see you next week, preferably on Friday.

Pt: What about my physical therapy?

Dr: I want to lay off that. I think physical therapy is very, very important in the treatment of backache, but I think you never had a good trial at bed rest.

Pt: No, because I was going to physical therapy.

Dr: The only time I want you up is to go to the bathroom, and I really don't want you sitting up in bed. Do you have a firm mattress?

Pt: Well, I haven't been able to get in bed since October.

Dr: Well, that's where I want you.

Pt: I have like a loveseat pull-out bed and it's low to the floor so I, my legs . . .

Dr: Well, then you need to get a board or something and put it under that sleeper.

Pt: It's like a board.

Dr: Okay, if it's very hard and firm that's good.

Pt: Okay, it's like that.

Dr: It doesn't sag anywhere . . .

Pt: No, it's straight, and it's real low to the floor.

Dr: Fine. That's where I want you then, other than going to the bathroom and eating your meals, flat on your back. Okay?

Pt: Now will you explain to me again what the Motrin is?

Dr: Motrin is an anti-inflammatory drug. It's an arthritic drug.

Pt: In other words, it's supposed to help the pain in the back.

Dr: A lot of the pain in back injuries is due to irritation of the tissues and this will quiet down that irritation of the tissues, that in conjunction with, first of all, the rest. I didn't feel too much muscle spasm in your back now.

Pt: Well, that has quieted down some. I had quite a bit in October. It sort of quit, but I still have the pain.

Dr: There's your prescriptions, here's the Darvocets, only take that as needed for extra pain. The Motrin I want you to take one, four times per day; breakfast, lunch, dinner, bed time and you should take that continuously . . . I want to see you next week, preferably on Friday, that will give us a full week. Okay? And we will see in a week, see how you are doing and, as I said, in the meantime, I'll review the x-rays. Okay? Anything else?

Pt: I wanted to mention to you. I had gone for a Pap smear and they said the Pap smear was normal, I mean I don't have cancer . . .

Notice how the physician shares his findings and clarifies the plan of action, including what he will do and what he expects the patient to do. Note, too, how the patient at the last minute brings up her concern about cancer possibly being the cause of her pain. The physician can now offer her appropriate reassurance that the etiology of her pain is not cancer; moreover, he will know that the patient's fear of cancer may reappear if the pain does not improve. It is not at all unusual for critical information like this to surface at the close of the interview when the patient feels comfortable and can see that she is being listened to. It is vital, therefore, that you demonstrate your open-ended attitude even as you close the encounter, as this physician did with his "Okay? Anything else?"

CHAPTER 7

Clinical Judgment in the Medical Interview

. . . To Ivan Ilych only one question was important: was his case serious or not? But the doctor ignored that inappropriate question. From his point of view it was not the one under consideration, the real question was to decide between a floating kidney, chronic catarrh or appendicitis. It was not a question of life or death, but one between a floating kidney and appendicitis.

Tolstoy, *The Death of Ivan Ilych*

Throughout the text we emphasize the use of the medical interview as a method of obtaining objective and precise data. Our main focus is the medical history as a diagnostic tool, but most interactions between doctors and patients are not purely diagnostic in nature. The data you obtain may be used to delineate other problems (not strictly defined as diseases) bearing on your patient's illness; they may serve as a starting point for patient education or may be used to assess your patient's progress or the outcome of therapy. We argue that most of the information you need to make diagnoses and take care of patients comes from your one-to-one interaction with the patient, the interview, and physical examination. In one sense, we stress completeness—the complete delineation and clarification of symptoms and dysfunction. However, there is another sense of "completeness" that is unattainable in a medical interview, a physical examination, or in any patient care situation, no matter how many diagnostic tests you use. **There is no such entity as a complete history and physical.**

Clinicians never have all the data that may be relevant to a given illness or disease situation or a given patient. There is always something left out, and all diagnostic and therapeutic decisions are made in the context of some uncertainty. We use various devices to minimize uncertainty but, in the long run, a physician usually acts to help his or her patient before the data are "complete." We make assumptions without knowing "for sure."

For example, we assume, based on past experience, based on our knowledge of the incidence of disease, that the 30-year-old man without gastrointestinal symptoms does not need a sigmoidoscopy. Can we say with 100 percent certainty that no abnormality would be found were we to do one? No. However, a good history is the most effective and efficient way to ensure that our assumption is correct. If we uncover an episode of rectal bleeding or a family history of intestinal polyposis, all bets are off. As Alvan Feinstein put it, all our diagnostic and therapeutic decisions are, in a sense, experiments; we formulate a hypothesis, change variables, and see what happens (Feinstein, 1967). We weigh probabilities, risks, benefits, experience, knowledge of pathophysiology, and opinions of our peers, but we are still left with hypotheses—perhaps well supported or perhaps more questionable—that have to be tested. Unfortunately, the experiments are complex ones involving humans in whom it is impossible to change one variable while keeping all others constant. Is this disease really causing the symptoms? Will this medication really help the patient? Learning to accept and work within this uncertainty is a major part of professional education for physicians. Sound **clinical judgment** is simply the logical and empathic approach to decision making in this context of uncertainty.

Figure 2 illustrates the feedback loop of clinical judgment as it occurs in a medical interview. Elements of process or technique allow the physician to obtain certain data (content), which ultimately must be organized into the traditional sections of a medical history (for instance, present illness, patient profile). But even the initial fragmentary content stimulates the clinician to formulate hypotheses, which then influence the continuing process of data collection. Figure 2 lists four different types of hypotheses that might be generated, as suggested by Platt and McMath (1979). Naturally, the overt concern of clinical practice relates to **differential diagnosis,** hypotheses about the disease from which the patient suffers. But differential diagnoses depend on more basic or preliminary hypotheses about the story itself: How does it fit together? Did X happen before or after Y? The effective clinican should, at the same time, be generating hypotheses about what sort of person the patient is: What sort of coping style does he or she have? What might one expect in terms of compliance or behavior change? Finally, there are hypotheses about the process of the interview itself: What is going wrong? Why do I feel so frustrated or uncomfortable? Chapters 8 and 9 consider hypotheses about the types of interviewing problems that arise when caring for "difficult" patients.

We consider in this chapter some topics raised by the uncertainty of doctor-patient interactions. First, we will discuss briefly the different types of error you will make in medicine and their relationship to the elusive "completeness" of our clinical activities such as interviewing. Second, we will consider what goes on inside your head as you conduct the interview. What drives your inquiries? Does the interview simply grow by ac-

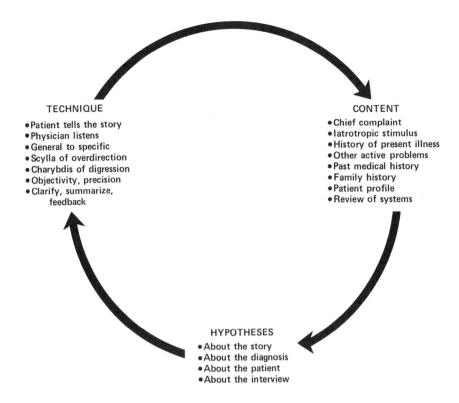

TECHNIQUE
• Patient tells the story
• Physician listens
• General to specific
• Scylla of overdirection
• Charybdis of digression
• Objectivity, precision
• Clarify, summarize,
    feedback

CONTENT
• Chief complaint
• Iatrotropic stimulus
• History of present illness
• Other active problems
• Past medical history
• Family history
• Patient profile
• Review of systems

HYPOTHESES
• About the story
• About the diagnosis
• About the patient
• About the interview

FIGURE 2. Feedback loop for the medical interview.

cretion, or does it change shape and move purposefully as it goes along and you test hypotheses? We will review some psychologic biases that make it difficult to think logically about the real probability of a given problem or diagnosis. Finally, we will list some heuristics for good problem solving in clinical interactions, with particular emphasis on problem solving within the medical interview. These are pragmatic guidelines, but the most significant of all guidelines is the rule that all guidelines have exceptions.

TYPES OF ERRORS

As medical students we make many errors in evaluating patients (Table 7); we continue to make errors as house officers and throughout our lives as practicing physicians. Some of these errors are avoidable, and some are not. **One kind of mistake** arises from your own lack of knowledge of what is known, or culpable ignorance. While it is impossible to command all medical knowledge, we each become thoroughly familiar with the medi-

TABLE 7. Types of Error in Medical Decisions

1. Clinician lacks knowledge of the subject matter.
2. Current state of medical knowledge is inadequate.
3. Biologic events are by nature probabilistic.
4. Clinician breaches the patient's trust.
5. Clinician uses faulty logic (intellectual error).

cal specialty in which we practice and continue to keep that knowledge up-to-date. However, regardless of how well informed you are, you will make some factual errors sometimes—because you are too busy with too many patients or because you are distracted by some other problem, and so forth. For example, you may be preoccupied with a dying patient with whom you have just had a difficult discussion about her desire for termination of life support. Your next patient has a relatively simple illness, a sore throat. You do a culture, and because you suspect streptococcus, you write out a prescription for penicillin for the patient to take pending the outcome of the culture. The patient informs you she is allergic to penicillin. You forgot to ask. So one kind of uncertainty in clinical interactions arises from your not knowing what you should know or forgetting it.

A **second error** arises from the state-of-the-science. We treated enlarged thymus glands with irradiation in the 1940s, threatened abortions with diethylstilbestrol in the 1950s, and upper respiratory infections with chloramphenicol in the 1960s. Each of these therapies was mistaken and actually posed a health risk that outweighed the benefits. Undoubtedly, we are making similar kinds of mistakes today that will only become clear to us when medical knowledge enlarges. In the interview we may emphasize the relationship of certain patient activities to the development, prevention, or treatment of disease; for example, diet as a way to prevent or treat coronary artery disease, or maternal alcohol usage and infant mental retardation. Yet each of these associations is controversial and will undoubtedly be clarified in the future.

A **third error** is based on the probabilistic nature of events in medicine and biologic variability. For example, since drugs affect different people differently, the best we can do is to say that we expect a high rate of cure or a low rate of side effects in a certain situation. But even when the probabilities clearly indicate that a decision is correct, the improbable may in fact occur, leading to an adverse effect. The natural history of a person's unique illness is not rigidly determined by the factors we understand. The second and third types of errors may well be related: with greater medical knowledge, fewer biologic events will appear to be probabilistic and more will be clearly determined by known factors. Whether this probabilistic error is ultimately reducible to state-of-the-science error is a philosophic question beyond the range of our discussion.

Breach of trust is a **fourth error** that occurs when we fail to obtain informed consent, or break the obligation requiring confidentiality. We are guilty of breach of trust when we lie to our patients or mislead them, when we blithely accept our version of their best interest without appropriate respect for their own wishes. While this type of error is subject matter for medical ethics, you make "ethical decisions" repeatedly in the interview. You avoid breach of trust in the interview by actively eliciting and listening to your patient's ideas and values regarding the illness and its management. Although there has been little critical study of precisely how one goes about the difficult task of discussing anticipated risks and benefits with patients, a good first step is listening.

The **fifth mistake** is a breakdown in thinking—intellectual error or faulty logic. Investigators concerned with decision making in medicine have focused primarily on this area and mostly on the part of it dealing with diagnosis: the making and testing of hypotheses in the process of diagnosis. Did you see the facts correctly? Did you judge what is probable in a given situation as well as what is possible? For example, if a patient complains of tarry stools you must logically use this fact to guide the interview and elicit other gastrointestinal symptoms that would help rule in or rule out upper GI bleeding as the cause.

Good interviewing skills help eliminate these errors in logic as you interact with patients. As you learn the basic knowledge and skills of how to conduct an adequate interview, you also learn to devise your interview strategy to move in a logical direction; the more open-ended the interview, the less you miss both facts and values.

Error and Completeness

Another way to categorize mistakes is to divide them into **errors of commission** and **errors of omission**. You can either **do** the wrong thing or **fail to do** the right one. These categories cut across the types of error listed previously. Factual mistakes, limitations of medical knowledge in general, breach of trust or faulty logic can all occur, both in actions that you take or actions that you fail to take. These concepts have important ramifications when we consider the completeness of our history taking and physical examination. We often talk of doing a medical test for the sake of completeness. It is one of those pat phrases that one hears daily on rounds. We have come to think of Completeness as something like "Big Brother," or perhaps as an unacknowledged entity that stalks our halls demanding daily sacrifices. We gaze furtively at one another, wondering what evil might befall us if we do not placate Completeness. We all do things "for completeness' sake" and, interestingly, such actions may lead to a paradoxic situation: our job is to help sick people, but often, insofar as we do things for completeness' sake, our actions are less likely to be done for the patient's sake.

All this is another way of saying that errors of commission are generally more sanctioned in medicine than errors of omission. You rarely get into trouble with your peers if you order extra studies or make the examination more complete than necessary, unless you order a very invasive and expensive test that is obviously unnecessary. On the other hand, you are frequently called on to justify yourself when you do not order a diagnostic test that may even be only mildly relevant to a particular illness, or that is relevant but unnecessary because its result will not change any therapeutic decision. We make decisions about completeness all the time when we interview patients. We may decide, for example, to forego the history of childhood diseases in the 85-year-old woman with hypertension or to skip the sexual history in a new patient who presents with acute back pain. One often feels, however, that the appropriateness of omitting certain parts of the history is less likely to be praised than the inappropriateness of a too "invasive" history is to be criticized. One continually weighs the value of the information likely to be obtained against the limits of the patient's tolerance to be interviewed, whether he or she is too sick or too tired or would feel that certain matters are too private.

Many physicians justify completeness by a call to "defensive medicine." They claim that they have to do a CT scan in a young man with a bumped head who never lost consciousness, because the case may end up in court some day. The issue of malpractice suits is one we cannot consider here, except to say that such suits most often arise when bad feelings are superimposed upon bad results. Most malpractice suits stem from poor communication, failure to obtain accurate and precise patient data, too little time spent explaining diagnoses or procedures, poor rapport, misunderstandings, and personality clashes. Good medical interviewing helps avoid all of these. Of course, good communication will not eliminate every threat of liability. And if you order enough tests defensively, for the sake of completeness, occasionally one will be truly useful. But how many errors of commission, with all their attendant costs and risks, will you have to make in order to prevent one serious error of omission? All the excessive studies and overtreatment performed in the name of completeness constitute an enormous chunk of professionally sanctioned "malpractice" that, at present, rarely ends up in court and is rarely discussed.

Defensive medicine aside, there are psychologic reasons why we tend to favor errors of commission. We are action oriented, we want to help the patient, we feel ourselves under pressure to **do something** to ease suffering, and we do not like to wallow in ambiguity. We view high-technology medicine as an exciting scientific accomplishment and ourselves as applying its benefits to sick people. It is not difficult to understand why we are less sensitized to possible errors of completeness (which is a kind of mottled thinking) and overtreatment (which may lead to iatrogenic illness) than we are to possible errors of not doing enough for our patient.

HYPOTHESES AND PROBABILITY IN THE INTERVIEW

Completeness obviously does not provide a sufficient guide for making diagnoses and prescribing therapy. Facts are not enough; you have to think. It is useful to consider what is actually going on in your head as you interview your new patient and take his or her medical history. Some of your preceptors will stress "completeness" as if there were a certain finite body of medical facts that, once obtained, would fit together like a jigsaw puzzle. You collect nondescript volumes of data and later, when you sit down to think about it, its meaning materializes. If you collect data in this fashion during the interview, you exhaust both yourself and the patient. Diagnosis does not occur in this way. In fact, one uses a **hypothetico-deductive** approach rather than an **inductive** one. In other words, you must constantly consider "guesses" or hypotheses, which you try to support or refute throughout the interview, physical examination, and subsequent diagnostic strategy.

Elstein and his co-workers at Michigan State University (1978) showed that experienced physicians generate a variety of hypotheses about what causes the patient's problem within the first two minutes, and often within the first 30 seconds, of the patient interaction. They found that data gathering is constantly changing its character based on what has gone before. They discovered that physicians have a fairly limited ability to juggle a variety of hypotheses that might explain a given problem, usually no more than five hypotheses at a time. Clinicians then design their questioning and other testing to obtain data that either supports one or more of the hypotheses, or tends to disprove or weigh against them. They continue this process until one hypothesis stands out sufficiently from the others to be acted on, or to permit the diagnosis to be made. Thus, the clinical method, just like the scientific method, does not involve gathering an enormous amount of data and then seeing how all the parts fit together later; rather, most data are collected for the purpose of testing hypotheses. For example, on the most elementary level, as soon as you walk into the room and see that the patient is a female of a particular race and age you know that some diagnoses are possible, while others are impossible.

The nature of this process means that **probability testing** is a major feature of clinical judgment within the interview as well as for therapeutic and diagnostic decisions. We ask questions most likely to clarify the problem and use the treatment most likely to help. Ideally, probability testing requires (1) a broad knowledge of pathophysiology and therapeutics; (2) prior probability (or prevalence) estimates for the given disease, based on textbook facts and, later, our own experience; and (3) a logical approach to estimating how probability changes. Good clinicians integrate these functions in making clinical judgments all the time, but they frequently find it difficult to dissect out the different elements of this process so that they can be stated clearly. Researchers in clinical judgment have discovered that we are all subject to certain psychologic biases that can distort our clinical thinking. Within the interview these biases distort our hearing and understanding of the patient's symptoms and change the strategy of our deductive approach in much the same way—albeit in the opposite direction—as sound logic. These biases might make a particular diagnosis feel more probable or less probable than it really is. While as human beings we are all subject to errors in judgment, we can minimize them by bringing them into the open and by understanding just what they are and how they occur.

Bias

Table 8 lists a number of such psychologic biases important in medicine. The bias of **availability** means that the doctor's assessment of how probable a diagnosis is relates to how easy it is for instances or occurrences of that disease to be brought to mind. This is simply another way of saying that the things that you are more familiar with, that you are more confident knowing about, tend to appear to be more likely than those that are more uncertain or obscure. A diagnosis might seem more probable than it really is, if you have seen a patient who proved to have a similar diagnosis last week, or if you have just been reading about that disease in your textbook. Within the interview, you might go right to a series of closed or leading questions to discover what you suspect on the basis of recent reading, thereby shutting out other symptoms that point to the real problem. For example, if you have just read the chapter on lymphomas, you may think that your patient with the chief complaint of "swollen glands" has Hodgkin's disease until proven otherwise. You may ask first about night sweats and weight loss, only later finding out that his 10-year-old son had a similar illness the previous week and that other symptoms suggest the much more likely simple infection.

In a similar way, a subspecialist is likely to perceive diseases in his or her subspecialty as occurring more frequently than they really do in the general population or among people with the same set of symptoms who go to primary care doctors. Gastroenterologists are more likely than other doctors to diagnose GI disease, not only because their patients tend, of course, to have clear-cut GI symptom complexes, but also because they overvalue GI diagnoses among patients who have symptom complexes that are also compatible with non-GI diagnoses.

TABLE 8. Psychologic Biases in Estimating Probability

1. Availability	4. Anchoring and adjustment
2. Representativeness	5. Rule-in favoritism
3. Sunk costs	6. Occam's razor

Representativeness is another frequent psychologic bias, particularly among physicians who stick closely to their textbooks and clinical literature. These doctors often think a rare disease is very probable if a patient has the representative or classic symptoms of that disease. Let us say a disease has five characteristic symptoms but is extremely rare, occurring in only one out of every million people. The five symptoms might be dizziness, right upper quadrant abdominal pain, frequent headaches, difficulty sleeping, and waking up in the morning with muscle stiffness. Each of these symptoms is quite common in itself. The fact that a patient has all five at once certainly makes him or her considerably more likely to have the rare disease; but more prevalent, ordinary diseases are still the most probable explanation for the patient's illness. Even though the patient provides a "representative" picture, other, common diseases are more likely to explain his or her problem than the rare disease. This does not mean that correct clinical judgment would never allow for making a very rare diagnosis, but it does mean that pursuing such a diagnosis usually has more to do with utility (see next section) than it does with probability. This is a common problem early in a physician's medical career, when he or she has little practical experience with the prevalence and incidence—or probability—of diseases. Every disease seems as likely as any other, every symptom is as likely to "represent" a rare disease as a common one.

If a certain amount of money or effort has already been invested in pursuing a given diagnostic strategy, the outcome or yield from that strategy may appear more likely than it really is, and the doctor may continue further tests so as not to "waste" those already performed. This is the bias called **sunk costs**. Let us say that a patient is ill with general muscle aching, malaise, and possible intermittent fevers. He also had some nonspecific abdominal pain that, when you first took the history, you believed was suggestive of gastrointestinal pathology. You then ordered an upper GI x-ray series (normal), and on subsequent discussion with the patient have found that the GI symptoms are really not as important a part of the syndrome as you first thought. The bias of sunk costs will tend to make you feel more compelled to complete the GI work-up, for example, with a barium enema and sigmoidoscopy, rather than to leave it "hanging."

In a very broad sense, the fact that you have a hypothesis, or several of them, tends to make you look more carefully at observations relevant to those hypotheses and to ignore other observations. You must have a frame of reference for your thinking. Clear thinking will necessarily lead more and more strongly in a given direction, simply because the remaining hypotheses are judged very probable or very useful or both. The bias of sunk costs is an exaggeration of this process, which leads to focusing too intently on a diagnosis simply because of your investment in it and then, perhaps, not being open to new data that may change your thinking.

Availability, representativeness, and sunk costs can be observed every day in the practice of medicine. The bias called **anchoring and adjustment** is a little more arcane. Doctors use some rough estimate of subjective probability to start with and then "anchor" their opinions at that level, using an adjustment factor to revise their opinion upward or downward as a result of new information. It is psychologically difficult to condense vast ranges of probability into the diagnostic problem frame, particularly since you know the patient is ill and there is a 100 percent probability that **something** is wrong. What can you do with a differential diagnosis in which one hypothesis has a 75 percent probability and another a 0.001 percent probability? Physicians cope with this problem by anchoring their estimates in a middle range, so that very unlikely diagnoses get overvalued and likely diagnoses often get undervalued. The adjustment factor after considering new evidence tends to be smaller in either direction than really warranted by the facts. The net effect is that judgments hover toward the middle level of probability and doctors often consider diseases that have vastly different likelihoods with only modestly different seriousness in pursuing their diagnostic strategy.

Since medicine demands action, there is also a bias in favor of making the diagnosis out of the array of hypotheses available. Elstein (1978) and other students of clinical decision making have found that physicians often seek out and evaluate evidence to support their main hypotheses but are less aggressive in seeking out evidence that could rule out this hypothesis. This tendency might be called **rule-in favoritism**. Within the interview, for example, you might actively seek symptoms such as nausea, radiation to the jaw or left arm, and sweating to support your hypothesis that the patient's chest pain is due to coronary insufficiency. You may not ask if the pain occurs with lying down or is relieved by antacids to try to rule out esophageal reflux. The worth of an open-ended question such as "Did you notice anything else?" is its power to elicit that datum we simply forgot or did not think of because of this bias.

We should also mention the tendency to try to make one diagnosis, rather than several. This is actually a reasonable clinical guideline, a heuristic that all students of medicine should take into consideration when evaluating the patient's history and physical findings. It is called **Occam's Razor**, named after William of Occam, a 14th century scholastic philosopher. In medicine this means that we should try to explain the entire illness—all the symptoms—with one diagnosis. While this is a good rule to keep in mind, it is certainly not always correct, especially in these days of multiple chronic and degenerative diseases. In particular, two common diseases (for example, diabetes mellitus and peptic ulcer) are much more likely as the explanation of a symptom complex of abdominal pain, vomiting, polyuria, polydipsia than is one rare disease (for example, acute intermittent porphyria). Occam's Razor supports the bias of representativeness when it makes us favor latching on to an uncommon diagnosis to avoid considering the less intellectually satisfying alternative of partitioning the illness among several explantions.

Utility and Clinical Judgment

Clinical judgment is conditioned by utility as well as probability. Diagnoses or decisions are not ends in themselves but tools for making the patient feel better. Thus, we want to pay particular attention to certain kinds of diagnostic hypotheses even when they are not judged to be very probable or the most probable explanation. For example, serious diseases (**seriousness**) must be considered and ruled out much more aggressively than mild or self-limited diseases. Even though a positive test for microscopic blood in the stool of a healthy, asymptomatic individual most likely will **not** indicate cancer, it is medically appropriate to do a thorough evaluation of the GI tract in someone with such an unexplained finding. Given the sensitivity and specificity of that test (for instance, the stool guaiac), the risk of cancer in a person with a single positive test may only be 5 percent, but only a poor physician would ignore that risk.

Treatability is another aspect of utility. There is no point in pursuing diagnosis for the sake of diagnosis unless it can have some benefit for the patient. The mere fact of our knowing the diagnosis and satisfying our own curiosity about what factors led to what outcomes may really have no value for the patient. Our decisions should be dictated by utility for the patient, not utility for us, unless the patient is enrolled in an experimental protocol after having given informed consent. There is no sense in doing a liver biopsy on an alcoholic patient who comes in to the hospital with abnormal liver function tests, once we have ascertained that the result will have nothing to do with the patient's subsequent management. The same patient may, in the future, have recurrent episodes of abdominal problems or abnormal liver function, which would lead us to question our hypothesis of alcoholic liver disease, and at that point perhaps a biopsy would be indicated. But even then the decision must be dictated by what is best for the patient. Our "need to know" is not necessarily best for the patient, even when the risks and costs of further tests are low, and particularly when they are high, as is usually the case in complex, invasive studies.

The patient's own assessment of utility should have paramount value, although physicians often have a major impact on the patient's beliefs about utility. We do not believe, as some ethical and legal commentators suggest, that all medical decisions can or should always be made entirely independently by the rational patient. In fact, sick people tend to trust their physicians and do not want to be burdened with multiple decisions, even when they are fully able to understand the general nature and consequences of the options. Investigators have found that informed consent, although espoused by most patients, is not so highly valued by them when faced with actual decisions about their own medical care (Lidz et al, 1983). Patients tend to rely on their doctor's advice, rather than thinking through all the alternatives, expecting fidelity in their relationship. But fidelity in this relationship depends on the physician's understanding of the patient. Within the interview physicians who help patients express their values and who allow them to ask questions will learn what facts, from an array of many, this particular patient needs to know to make a decision. Consideration of the patient's own value system and decisions about whether or not to accept medical care is beyond the scope of this text but certainly has an impact on the questions of compliance and negotiation, which will be considered in Chapter 10.

HEURISTICS FOR THE MEDICAL INTERVIEW

We have adapted a set of guidelines for clinical judgment from the heuristics presented by Elstein, Schulman, and Sprafka (1978). These are an attempt to give you a "handle" or set of thinking skills to use as you proceed through your patient interview and physical examination; they are also useful, as you continue further, to judge strategies for diagnosis and management.

1. **Multiple, competing hypotheses.** You should think of a number of diagnostic possibilities compatible with the chief complaint and data obtained in the early part of the medical interview. Avoid making "snap" diagnoses, as this tends to make it difficult for you to hear data that suggest other etiologies.
2. **Probability.** Consider the most common diagnoses first.
3. **Utility.** Consider more seriously those diagnoses for which effective therapies are available, or for which treatment would be significantly different than that for competing diagnoses, and in which failure to treat would hurt the patient (that is, be a serious omission). Try to keep your estimates of the probability of a disease and the utility of diagnosing it separate.
4. **Branch and screen.** History taking and the physical examination should be branching procedures. You should develop screening tactics to avoid overly detailed examinations when unnecessary.
5. **Precision.** Strive for the degree of precision or reliability needed for the decision at hand. More than that is not necessary. For example, for many adult patients it is not necessary to know the fine details of every childhood illness; if, however, a patient states she had rheumatic fever as a child you must elicit historic evidence in support of the diagnosis, because that illness may have long-term consequences into adulthood.

6. **Plan.** Form a reasoned plan to test your hypotheses. There should be a reason for every datum you plan to gather.
7. **Disconfirmatory evidence.** Actively seek out and evaluate evidence that tends to rule out any hypothesis or action alternative, as well as the evidence that tends to confirm it.
8. **Multiple symptoms.** Consider the possibility that a patient with multiple symptoms or complaints may well have more than one disease.
9. **Harm versus benefit.** Consider what harm each test you order might do (and also its cost), as well as the benefits it might generate. In addition, do not order tests whose results will not logically make a difference in your decision-making process.
10. **Revision.** Continually revise probabilities as you collect more data.

CHAPTER 8

The Difficult Interview, Part 1: Technical, Process, and Topical Problems

. . . Seal up the mouth of outrage for a while
Till we can clear these ambiguities
And know their spring, their head, their true descent . . .

The Prince, *Romeo and Juliet*, Act V, Scene 3.

Our interactive model of the medical interview demands that both doctor and patient play an active role in generating "good data" that are as accurate and precise as possible. Sometimes even a novice interviewer finds it easy to get good data: the patient is alert, helpful, to the point, spontaneously brings up symptoms that the interviewer might not think to ask, the problem itself is relatively straightforward, and there are no awkward elements such as a sexual problem. Sometimes, however, the interviewer—and usually the patient also—becomes aware that things are not going well. We label particular patients or specific situations "difficult" when they present problems for us. These problems might arise from the patient, from the doctor, from the topic under consideration, or from extraneous events that are happening at the time. We have argued earlier in this book that **observer bias** and **instrument precision** play a part in any medical observation, whether they be gallium scans, auscultation of heart murmurs, or the recording of a medical history. There are ways of improving the quality of each of these observations even in the presence of adverse circumstances. For example, one might close the window in the room so that one can hear the heart murmur better, or jiggle the earpieces of the stethoscope to improve the air conduction component of perceiving a murmur. The same thing is true with the difficult patient situation; there are remedial actions to improve the outcome.

Although there are many variations on what can go wrong in an interview, we propose a simplified taxonomy of problems to help diagnose and

114

remedy specific difficulties that arise regularly no matter how expert the interviewer. These problems can happen to any physician and any patient at any time and are neither indication of failure nor cause for despair; in fact, overcoming these difficulties can be an exhilarating experience for both patient and physician. At times, however, when the difficulty is more than a matter of one interview, but pervades the entire doctor-patient relationship, it may be helpful to seek the advice of a colleague or suggest that a colleague assume the patient's care. It is useful to categorize difficult patient interactions into four general types, even though there is frequently overlap between or among them. These categories are listed in Table 9.

Technical or process problems include those occurring with delirious, foreign-speaking, or incompetent patients, or patients whose conversational style—reticent, rambling, vague—interferes with information ex-

---

TABLE 9. Difficult Patient-Doctor Interactions

A. Technical or Process Problems
    Technical impairments
        Organic (delirium, dementia)
        Language barrier
    Style impairments
        Reticence
        Rambling
        Vagueness
B. Topical Problems
    Drugs and alcohol
    Sexual history
    Positive ROS
C. Personality Styles (from Kahana and Bibring, 1964)
    Dependent, demanding patient
    Orderly, controlled patient
    Dramatizing, manipulative patient
    Long-suffering, masochistic patient
    Guarded, paranoid patient
    Superior patient
D. Somatization Disorders
E. Difficult Feelings and Defenses
    The patient's feelings and defenses
        Anxiety
        Anger
        Depression
        Denial
        Manipulation and Seductiveness
    The doctor's feelings and defenses

change. **Topical problems** arise with certain subject matter that may be difficult for the patient or the doctor to discuss. The patient's sexual history often presents such a problem, one that might require particular sensitivity and skill on the part of the interviewer. Patients are also sometimes reluctant to discuss drug and alcohol usage, previous medical care contacts, or alternate forms of health care, such as visits to a chiropractor or the use of health foods and fad diets. Technical problems tend to be global impediments to information gathering; topical problems are more localized to a specific time or topic.

While technical and topical problems arise in "ordinary" medical interviews, other problems arise when the patient's (or the doctor's) personality style or affective state (or both) become major issues in managing a patient's medical condition. We will discuss these problems in Chapter 9.

DIFFICULT PROCESS

Technical Impairments

One type of difficult interview occurs when there are technical problems with obtaining information from the patient. Obvious examples are when the patient speaks another language or is comatose or semicomatose, delirious, psychotic, or demented. The patient simply lacks the cognitive or language skills to give good historic information that the physician can understand. Here are two examples of technical problems, the first a non-English–speaking patient and the second an elderly, demented patient.

In this interview with an Iranian woman, everything went along pretty well until the physician asked the patient if she had any allergies:

> Dr: And do you have cough? *(demonstrates)*
> Pt: No, no cough.
> Dr: Fever? Hot? *(touches forehead)*
> Pt: Yes, yes I feel hot.
> Dr: Uh, allergy to medicine? Pill give you rash? Reaction? *(points all over skin, scratching to get at idea of itchy rash)*
> Pt: *(Looking confused)* I don't know.
> Dr: Excuse me, I'll get your brother to help us speak.

In the following encounter with an elderly, demented patient, the patient simply cannot remember the symptoms he has been experiencing; rather, he is only aware of how he feels at present:

> Dr: Do you know who I am?
> Pt: Well, I don't know, no.
> Dr: I'm Dr. Smith.

Pt: Oh.

Dr: I'm glad to see you today. How have you been feeling?

Pt: Oh, I don't know, just all poured out.

Dr: Weak, are you weak?

Pt: I imagine to a certain extent, but it seems just that nothing just seems to be right.

Dr: *(Taking pulse)* Your pulse feels good today.

Pt: I'm glad there's something good about me.

Dr: Do you feel there's not much good about you?

Pt: Oh well, I guess I'm just average.

Dr: How's your heart been treating you?

Pt: Oh, it never did bother me.

Dr: How are you sleeping at night?

Pt: No trouble at all.

Dr: How's your appetite?

Pt: Always with me.

We do not ordinarily label these situations "difficult," because we quickly dismiss the possibility of a useful interview and seek information elsewhere. In our examples, the physician got an interpreter for the Iranian woman and interviewed a family member of the demented patient. In fact, the elderly gentleman's wife stated that his appetite was poor, that he was having trouble sleeping, and that he was frequently short of breath.

There are other situations, however, that present problems of a more subtle—and more frustrating—nature. The profoundly depressed patient may not have enough energy to give a detailed, logical story of his problem; the anxious and talkative patient may embellish her story with unnecessary details. Some patients are so reticent that you find yourself asking closed question after closed question until the interview comes to a distressing stop; others seem to have so much to say that you feel as though you are losing control, getting confused about what the diagnosis is, and worried that when the time is up you may know a lot about the patient but very little about the illness. Let us look at ways to handle some of these problems; in particular, we will look at the reticent patient, the patient who rambles, and the vague patient. In each instance we will try to define the problem, give examples, and suggest possible remedies.

Style Impairments

THE RETICENT PATIENT

The Problem. The reticent patient is the patient who does not say enough. Sometimes this is no problem and may even be desirable; for example, the young person with a simple complaint like a sore throat in which only a limited amount of information is needed to develop a diagnostic strategy or therapeutic plan of action; or the patient with uncomplicated acute trauma such as a laceration. There are other times, however, when the lack of detail in a history creates serious problems in establishing the etiology of a symptom; for example, the patient with chest pain in whom a detailed and unambiguous history is essential for making the diagnosis. Such a patient may be very willing to answer "yes" or "no" and you soon find yourself asking question after question in very tedious fashion and then running out of questions before gaining any idea as to what is going on.

The Remedy. Here the trick is to guide the patient without asking leading questions; sometimes one way of asking an open-ended question works when another way does not. Consider this example:

> Dr: Can you tell me what the problem is?
> Pt: Uh, that's what I came to see you about, Doc.
> Dr: What have your symptoms been?
> Pt: Tired, awful tired.

It almost appears as though the interview will come to a dead stop with the first question, but the interviewer simply asks another open-ended question that this time around elicits the chief complaint.

Another trick is to use a menu. This interview went on:

> Dr: Can you tell me more about it?
> Pt: No, just tired.
> Dr: When you say tired, do you mean a feeling of not being rested or a feeling of weakness in your muscles? Or do you have trouble doing things you used to do because you get short of breath?
> Pt: That's it, Doc, just not rested.

The physician uses a menu or "laundry list" to clarify further the symptom without leading the patient. Notice the difference between asking the patient to make a choice of a response and asking the same questions in sequence in yes/no fashion. If you find yourself asking many yes/no questions, you should evaluate the worth of the response. The data are better when patients volunteer information than when the information has to be elicited, because in the latter instance, you can never be sure that these patients are not simply being agreeable or saying what they think they should say.

There are many reasons why some patients do not say much. Some of the more common ones are depression, dementia (the patient simply cannot remember his or her symptoms), anxiety, and denial. Some patients expect to be interrogated like witnesses and must learn that we value their own selection and sequence of responses. These persons may have trouble with a directive such as "Tell me what happened," but may do better with "Tell me what happened first" and then "What happened next?" and even better with frequent reminders demonstrating your open, relaxed attitude that "It is important to know exactly how you felt when that happened— tell me as best you can . . ."

THE PATIENT WHO RAMBLES

The Problem. Some patients embellish their problems with numerous details that seem unrelated to the reason they came to see the doctor. In other settings such patients might be considered exquisite storytellers, but you may have a limited amount of time in which to get the story and you do not wish to be entertained. Sometimes the details seem connected to the story; at other times it is difficult to see any connection at all. Sometimes the details are all part of the medical history, but there are too many of them all at once; at other times the details are unnecessary, such as the patient who has an attack of diarrhea and describes in great detail his or her attempt to find a bathroom.

The Remedy. Here the trick is to direct the patient back to the task at hand without appearing to be rude or uninterested. One way to do this is to acknowledge one's own confusion and feeling of being lost in the details, as well as one's need to accomplish the task in a limited period of time. Most patients accept this kind of direction very well. For example, you might say to the patient with diarrhea:

> Dr: It certainly sounds as though you had a hard time with that episode; since our time is limited, perhaps you can tell me more about the diarrhea itself. Have you ever had this problem before?

In this instance, the physician uses a summary statement ("sounds as though you had a hard time . . ."), a reminder of time constraints, followed by a question that directs the interview back to the diarrhea, all the while making it clear that he or she is interested in what the patient has to say.

Here is an example, similar to one presented in Chapter 3, of an open-ended question that leads to a deluge of disconnected information that would leave most students and many physicians feeling totally bewildered:

> Dr: Now what can I do for you, Mrs. P?
>
> Pt: Well, first of all, I'm here mainly because I've been experiencing that tired, worn-out feeling, most of the time. I can go to bed say 9:00 in the evening and get up at 8:00 or even later and I still feel very tired. And, I don't know, maybe that's due, I've been still experiencing hot flashes and sometimes now it's not, I don't experience them as often as I used to but I still do and especially towards the evening or at night, and it awakens me when I do experience something like that. Maybe that's part of the reason why I feel so tired, I don't know. Anyways, now in the evening when I experience this kind of a hot feeling I just get that craving I want to eat, you know, or sometimes it works just the opposite where I feel kind of nervous, I get that nervous feeling, and now last week I had headaches just about every day on arising . . .

Although this patient may have just stated most of her medical history, it is hard to sort out each bit of data. The fear most of us have of asking open-ended questions is that we may receive precisely this kind of rambling response. In reality, such responses occur infrequently. The best thing to do is to acknowledge your confusion and try to direct the patient to one topic at a time. One possible reply might be:

> Dr: Okay, I'm getting a bit confused. Let's see if we can take one problem at a time. You mentioned tiredness even though you seem to get a lot of sleep. Other than the hot flahes, is there anything else that seems to wake you up at night?

Either during or after the interview, you will have a chance to think about why the patient talks this way. There are many possible etiologies, among them anxiety, loneliness, thought disorder, or the relationship between an event (described in seemingly unnecessary detail) and a symptom or a belief about a symptom. Sometimes this kind of response is simply the person's conversational style, which seems less appropriate when used in a professional relationship than in a social interaction; sometimes the associations are so bizarre and the rambling so severe that you must consider psychiatric illness as the cause.

THE VAGUE PATIENT

The Problem. With this type of patient, the interviewer cannot figure out exactly what the patient is describing. You may wonder whether it is the symptom that is vague or the patient's description that is vague. Some sensations are rather difficult for people to describe; for example, dizziness or poorly localized abdominal pain. This is particularly frustrating when the diagnosis rests principally on an unambiguous history, as in the case of angina, migraine, or vertigo. When you have known the patient before, it is easier to know whether the problem is with the patient's description or with the symptom itself; the patient who has always given a precise history and is unable to describe a symptom precisely is probably experiencing a vague symptom, whereas a patient who has always given a vague history may well have a precise symptom that simply requires more work to translate into words that mean something to the physician.

The Remedy. Here the technique is to give the patient a choice of words that mean something to you, but without leading the patient. For example, you might use a menu such as "Was the pain sharp or dull?" and "Was it all over or in one place or did it move from place to place?" Or you can ask if it is anything like a symptom with which both patient and physician are familiar, such as (for lower abdominal or pelvic pain in a woman) "Does it feel anything like menstrual cramps?" Another approach is to ask the patient if he or she has ever felt anything like this particular symptom before, and then to ask, "What's different about it this time?" To find the location of a vague symptom, you can point to various parts of the patient's body, especially while doing the physical examination, and ask, "Is this where it hurts?"

The following two examples illustrate vague patient openings. In the first, the doctor simply indicates that she will not accept vague terminology like "cold or flu" ("tell me more about what you mean") and the patient begins to describe his symptoms in more detail. The patient in the second example does not respond to simple requests for more precision. Here is the first example, in which the doctor helps the patient to be more precise:

Dr: What can I do for you?
Pt: *(Clears throat)* I think I've got, um, a cold or flu or something . . . yesterday I felt terrible, so I feel I just need some kind of a prescription . . .
Dr: Okay. Tell me, you say you have a cold, tell me more about what you mean.
Pt: Um *(clears throat)*, fatigue is the most . . .
Dr: Fatigue?
Pt: Just kind of drained.
Dr: Aha.
Pt: Kind of scratchy throat, not really sore. Ah, a lot of drainage . . .
Dr: Coughing?
Pt: A little bit, but not getting anything up.

> Dr: Just sort of dry?
>
> Pt: Dry coughing, I don't feel as though there's anything collected down here yet. And, that's another thing that worries me, having had a history of asthma, I have a fear of bronchitis.

Here is the second example, in which the patient's description remains vague:

> Pt: Well, doctor, well, I got the dizziness, I'm getting more, looks like I'm, looks like I'm getting tired and tired-er, I go up the steps and I just, just like dizziness, I, I go like this, I just go dark, I, and I can't see.
>
> Dr: What do you mean by dizziness?
>
> Pt: When I go up the steps and when I get up in the morning, I got that dizziness again, I'm just falling back.
>
> Dr: What happens to you when you're dizzy?
>
> Pt: Well, when, when I drink water, if I drink cold water, that's when I get it, then I start having chills, I get real cold, just like I'm shaking.
>
> Dr: But how do you feel when you're dizzy?
>
> Pt: I just go back, like this, and then sometime I, I can't see, I, I have to close my eyes like that and then open my eyes up like that and I still can't just like . . .

We are still left wondering whether the patient's description is vague or the symptom is vague. Dizziness is often hard for patients (even "precise" patients) to define. One remedy is to suggest a menu:

> Dr: When you say dizziness, is it a feeling that you may pass out or that you may lose your balance?
>
> Pt: No, not exactly.
>
> Dr: Could you describe it as a spinning sensation as though you or the room is moving, or is it more of a lightheadedness?
>
> Pt: That's it, lightheaded, just lightheaded.

While it would have been better for the patient to volunteer this information, you can be fairly safe in assuming that the patient does not have vertigo or presyncope.

Storytelling

All patients—whether reticent, verbose, rambling, or vague—are being asked for a story. You want a story that is clear, internally consistent, logical, and not fictional. Most patients desire these features as well but may not necessarily share with the physician the same criteria for judging them as such. Your first approach is to clarify and educate, teach or demonstrate the kind of story that will be helpful. If this approach does not work, you are probably faced with one of three problems: (1) the patient's basic personality style, perhaps stressed by the illness, interferes with telling an adequate story; (2) some strong emotion or affect gets in the way of the patient's telling a clear, logical story; or (3) the patient's beliefs are both different from yours and unspoken, so that a story that appears incoherent is actually quite logical, once one understands the basic premises from which the patient reasons.

We will examine these issues in Chapters 9 and 10. However, first we will consider the second category in our taxonomy, topical problems in the interview.

DIFFICULT TOPICS IN THE INTERVIEW

At times, it is not so much that there is a technical impediment to communicating with the patient, but rather that there is a specific topic that is difficult to talk about. In this section we will deal with three such topics: drug and alcohol use, the sexual history, and the "positive" review of systems. Each of these items is difficult for different reasons. A history of drug or alcohol abuse requires the patient to be truthful about something that he or she may wish to hide; the sexual history may violate certain taboos in our society of what constitutes proper material for conversation; the "positive" review of systems is tedious and overwhelming for both patient and physician.

Drug and Alcohol Use

The history of drug or alcohol use forces one to encounter a fundamental issue in medical interviewing, that of truth telling. Is the patient telling the truth? How does one judge intent? While physicians sometimes doubt the accuracy of patient reports, this is usually inappropriate as the patient is almost always the best witness of his or her own symptoms. The case may be different, however, with self-reports about certain kinds of behavior. The question of truthfulness is a common problem when trying to elicit dietary, smoking, drug, and alcohol histories. These are loaded areas, and most people (patients and physicians) feel that there are "right" answers and "wrong" answers to questions posed during the medical interview. For example, when asked "How much do you smoke?" many smokers reply "Too much." There is no quantification in this answer. The reply is colored by the patient's awareness that it is "wrong" to smoke. It may be easier for such patients to talk more neutrally about what age they started to smoke or how many times they have tried to quit.

Here is a smoking history obtained from a 40-year-old black man presenting with shortness of breath. The physician tries to find out exactly how much is "not too much" and also tries to determine the prior history of smoking in order to determine whether the patient's current respiratory symptoms caused him to cut down and also whether the cumulative smoking history is enough to cause certain respiratory illnesses, such as chronic bronchitis or carcinoma of the lung.

Dr: Okay. How much do you smoke?
Pt: Oh, not too much.
Dr: How much is not too much?
Pt: Oh, umm, not half a pack a day.
Dr: Is that as much as you've always smoked? Have you ever smoked more than that?
Pt: Uh, when I was barbering, I would smoke more, sometimes a pack. You know, but they would burn out. You know, because when I was doin' a customer or something, they'd burn out, so I'd just light up another one.
Dr: Uh hmm. How old were you when you started?
Pt: Thirteen.

Similarly, a dependence on drugs or alcohol is seen by most patients as a habit of which the physician will disapprove and some will deny the use of these substances, particularly if asked a yes/no question. Here is an example of a physician (who can smell the alcohol on the patient's breath) trying to elicit the history of alcohol use in a 28-year-old woman presenting for evaluation of hypertension:

Dr: You are using some aspirin and Tylenol?
Pt: Every once in a while. It's not regular but that's the only drugs I take.
Dr: And are you a pretty steady drinker?
Pt: I have one or two drinks at work, you know. After work I . . .
Dr: . . . Okay. Do you have any more than that?
Pt: Sometimes it's more than that but basically . . .
Dr: Is that something that would be hard for you to give up?
Pt: Well it's a very social type thing for me, I guess . . . so . . . ye, yeah, I'd have to think about it, ha ha.

Often in this situation it is not so much what the patient says but how she says it. This patient paused and looked away when asked about how much she drinks, and she began to use phrases such as "you know" and hedges such as "basically." She also displayed some nervous laughter. There are often such clues to the fact that the patient is saying something less than the truth; there may be pauses (time to censor material), shifts in position, eye aversion, and hedges in the verbalization, such as "not really" instead of "no." In this example, the physician does not gain much quantitative data about how much the patient actually drinks. The most revealing question is the indirect one ("Is that something that would be hard for you to give up?"), to which the patient's answer ranges from denial ("Well it's a very social type thing" to agreement ("I guess so, yeah") to ambivalence ("I'd have to think about it"). It is rarely useful to state to the patient that you doubt the accuracy of a story, especially when you have not already built a relationship with that person. You should, however, make a mental note of the behavior in the hope that at some time in the future you will be able to use the information to help the patient.

A Digression on the Question of Reliability

There are other times when you may doubt the accuracy of a patient's story; certainly you wonder about the reliability of patients with cognitive disorders or memory disorders who simply cannot remember their symptoms. Sometimes patients tell us things that we know to be erroneous. Here is an example of a patient reporting to her physician the results of blood pressure readings taken at a community screening:

Dr: Now Friday you had told me over the phone you had your blood pressure checked.

Pt: Yes.

Dr: At the mall. And they told you it was very high.

Pt: I told them all, I'm going to the doctor, I do have high blood pressure so I was going to bypass it and they insisted. So when she took it the first time it was a hundred and ninety-something over 180.

Dr: Mm hmm.

Pt: So they took it three times. The second time it was 200 over 193. A hundred and eighty or ninety or something. The last time it was 193 over a hundred and eighty-something.

Dr: Mm hmm. Your blood pressure today is 140 over 90, which is fine.

The blood pressure values this patient reports are clearly wrong and probably impossible. The issue, however, is not numbers, but rather the patient's anxiety. Notice that the physician neither confirms nor denies the accuracy of the patient's report but instead reassures the patient by bringing her back to the present and the currently normal state of her blood pressure. At other times one may want to "correct" the error by educating the patient as to the ranges usually found in blood pressure readings. The discussion might go something like this:

> Dr: Gee, those are interesting blood pressure readings. It sounds as though the upper readings may be right, but I'm not sure about the lower readings. You say 193 over 180? You know the two numbers that we usually give for a blood pressure, see, here's what yours usually look like *(demonstrates in patient's chart)*. Yours usually runs 160 over 100 or 140 over 92; once you went up to 180 over 100. But that lower number is always a lot less than the upper number even when your blood pressure is acting up. So I'm not sure if those numbers they gave you are correct. In any case, your blood pressure today is 140 over 90, which is fine.

The Sexual History

This is a normal part of the medical history. Depression, anxiety, and anger may relate to underlying sexual problems; conversely, many physical symptoms or diseases may lead to sexual dysfunction. Asking even a few questions about sexual functioning sends the message that the physician is willing and available to discuss sexual concerns if the patient wishes.

As with any other part of the medical interview, how much you need to know depends on the situation. There is no requirement to get a "complete" sexual history from every patient, just as there is no need to get a "complete" cardiorespiratory history from a 20-year-old woman who jogs six miles a day, has no shortness of breath, and has come for a pre-employment examination. While the sexual history is a regular part of the medical interview, sometimes one question ("Are you having any sexual problems?") suffices. If the patient answers in the negative, no more need be said at that point; you have, however, indicated that sexual problems are legitimate fare for discussion to which the patient may return later (either in that visit or a subsequent one). Of course, some patients will answer a simple screening question about sexual problems in the affirmative. Then it is your job to be skillful and appear comfortable (even if you are not) in discussing sexual problems.

A discussion of sexual matters may not feel routine to the patient and may be unexpected, especially if the patient is used to physicians who do not ask about sex or if the patient feels he or she has a problem that is unrelated to sexual functioning. For example, the young man presenting with a severe sore throat may be very surprised at your interest in his sexual activity, unless you explain that his negative strep culture, negative test for mononucleosis, and his failure to improve raise the question of pharyngeal gonorrhea.

Unless it is the presenting complaint, one does not jump right in with sexual questions early in the interview. In fact, knowing something about the patient as a person facilitates asking questions that are always difficult. For example, once you know whether the patient is married or is living with someone, it is easier to ask about sexual preference and activity. When in doubt, you should use the term "partner" rather than a gender-specific term such as "boyfriend" or "wife." If you ask only about opposite-sex partners, the patient may infer that you would be shocked by a report of homosexual activity. The homosexual patient may, therefore, avoid relating his or her actual sexual preference. On the other hand, the happily married 65-year-old may well be offended by the use of the term "partner." There is no easy way to ask about sexual preference, but it is often necessary to know; the more you know about the patient's lifestyle, the easier it is to ask such intimate questions.

Delaying this part of the history until later in the interview will also make it easier to use words that the patient can understand, as you become more familiar with the patient's language style. As with other intimate bodily functions (voiding, defecating), patients may describe their sexual functioning with words that depend on their age, level of education, and cultural background; some descriptions may be idiosyncratic and obscure. If you listen for how each patient uses certain words, you find that "relationship" may be used to mean "sexual relationship," that "birth control" may be taken to mean oral contraceptives, and that "careful" (as in "being careful") to describe how the patient avoids pregnancy has numerous meanings. Open-ended questions permit the patient to use his or her own words; in your follow-up questions, you can use the patient's words, thereby ensuring a common language, once you know precisely what the patient's words mean.

The sexual history can be included in a nonthreatening way as part of the ROS, while dealing with menstrual or obstetric questions in women or with genitourinary questions in men. The focus is always on the patient's own perception of whether or not there is a sexual problem, not a voyeuristic account of frequency and techniques. As in any other intimate matter, you should not probe if the patient does not wish to discuss. You may continue with questions about other aspects of the health history, at the same time building rapport, returning to the sexual history if necessary when more trust exists.

Open-ended questions about sexual activity are preferable to closed questions. An open-ended question allows the patient to say as much or as little as he or she wishes. It also demonstrates that you are not interested only in a particular symptom or problem, but in the total person. Direct, very specific questions elicit less information and are not helpful in making the patient feel comfortable with this part of the medical history. Here are some examples of useful questions:

Are you having any sexual problems?

Do you have any questions or concerns about sexuality or sexual functioning?

Many people who are ill experience a change in their sexual function. Have you noticed any change?

Has your interest in sex changed recently? Since you've been ill? Since you've been on the new medicine for your blood pressure?

An introductory statement followed by a question often puts patients at ease:

A lot of men have sexual problems when they take Aldomet. Have you noticed any problems?

It sounds as though your marriage has been a good one. How about your sexual relationship?

Many girls your age have questions about sex and birth control. How about you?

If the patient answers these questions in such a way as to indicate problem areas, then more detailed questioning could be beneficial. Sexual dysfunction may result from physical, pharmacologic, or emotional problems, or any combination of the three. Physicians explore the medical reasons that may account for or contribute to dysfunction, as well as assess the emotional component.

The sexual history, like any other part of the medical interview, is focused to produce information appropriate to the situation. The history is more extensive when a patient requests birth control or fears a sexually transmitted disease, or when a sexual problem is the presenting complaint. Consider this example:

Dr: You don't look as tired as you were before.
Pt: I'm not as tired since I've been taking the iron.
Dr: That's helped, huh. Well, do you have another problem?
Pt: Yeah, with my stomach. When I have sex, my stomach hurts right here. After that, it doesn't bother me.
Dr: When you have sex? Otherwise you feel good?
Pt: Uh huh.
Dr: Okay. When did all this start?
Pt: About a month ago.
Dr: And has it gotten any better since that time?
Pt: Uh uh, it's the same.
Dr: Has it gotten any worse?
Pt: Sometimes it gets worse.
Dr: When you're not having sex you feel fine?
Pt: Uh huh. But sometimes, when I walk I get this real sore pain and then I get real bad.

Dr: When you have the pain during intercourse, is it all the time during intercourse or at the beginning or at the end? Or only when he is thrusting inside?
Pt: Right here.
Dr: Only on that side. Does it hurt anywhere else?
Pt: Uh uh.
Dr: Have you ever had this problem before?
Pt: It always did that.
Dr: So you've had this a long time.
Pt: Ah ha.
Dr: What made you think now it might be serious even though it didn't get worse?
Pt: It gets worse sometimes. But I just get . . . but I just thought it was nothing.
Dr: Can you think of any reason why you want to get it checked now?

Pain on intercourse can be a sign of pelvic pathology (pelvic inflammatory disease or endometriosis) or may be an expression of underlying depression or problems in the particular relationship. The physician in our example above follows the simple rules of good history taking, asking open-ended questions ("Do you have another problem?") and then the basic "when" ("When did all this start?"), "where" ("Does it hurt anywhere else?"), "why," and "why now" ("Can you think of any reason why you want to get it checked now?"). The physician follows up with more specific questions to obtain precise details of the problem ("When you have the pain during intercourse, is it all the time during intercourse or at the beginning or at the end? Or only when he is thrusting inside?") Because many patients have difficulty discussing such details, in part because they are unsure of what words are acceptable, the physician gives the patient a number of choices from which to choose her answer. This reticent patient has difficulty even with these choices and, instead, answers the question by pointing to the location of pain. The physician obtains the useful information that the pain is limited to one side.

In this example, because the symptom relates directly to sexual activity, there is much more that we need to know. It would be helpful to know if the patient's desire—libido—has changed ("Do you feel like making love—having sex—more or less than you used to?") or if her ability to enjoy sex has changed ("Do you feel satisfied when you make love?") Choose words that you are comfortable with and that the patient can understand. If you are not sure you are being understood, ask ("Do you understand what I am asking?"). As much as possible, you should ask questions that permit the patient to answer from her own point of view and in her own way ("Do you feel satisfied?" as opposed to "Do you have an orgasm?").

When you suspect a sexually transmitted disease it may be necessary to know sexual preference and numbers and regularity of sexual partners, and to ask if partners have had any sexually transmitted disease symptoms. These are always difficult questions to ask, because no one wants to have a sexually transmitted disease nor to acknowledge that a partner may have gone outside the relationship. Patients feel anger and guilt and may find the physician accusatory.

Skill is required to express your questions in the same neutral way that you talk about illnesses or infections: "Are you concerned that you might have gotten this from someone?" or "Is there any chance that you have been exposed to someone with a similar infection?" Such questions often help the patient talk about the situation more easily with responses such as "I don't see how I could have gotten this from my boyfriend unless he's not playing straight, while I am" or "My lover did go to the doctor because he had a drip but he never told me to get checked or anything." Sometimes it helps to introduce a difficult question with a statement, such as "I think you may have an infection that one can acquire only during intercourse, but I don't want to make any assumptions about your sexual relationships. Is it possible that you've been with someone who has this?" If the patient says "That's impossible," you must accept that statement as representing the patient's belief and best adaptation to the situation at that moment. The doctor can still prescribe the appropriate treatment and add "If you do know anybody who might have this, it would be good if you could tell them to get checked." Do not argue with the patient. If the diagnosis is uncertain, say so and outline the plan for making the diagnosis clear. In the case of reportable venereal diseases for which health departments do case finding, the doctor can say, "By law, I am required to report this illness, and there may be someone from the health department who will talk to you about who else might have it."

Another difficult situation arises with teenagers. Sexually active teens are at risk for sexually transmitted disease, and females, of course, are at risk for pregnancy. In evaluating any genitourinary or pelvic problem, it is therefore necessary to ask about sexual activity. You should do so, however, without implying either approval or disapproval of the patient's having intercourse. Some 13-year-old girls have been pregnant, while others have little knowledge of sexuality at all. It is helpful to begin with the patient's interest in school, social activities, then "boys" (or "girls"), and finally "sex." Some helpful questions are "Do you have any questions about your body? About sex? About how not to get pregnant?" or "Do you have any need for birth control?" or "Are your friends or the kids at school into having sex yet? How about you?" or "Some girls your age get pretty serious about boys and start having sex. How about you?" Patients should be allowed to answer in their own way, with your assurance that this information will be confidential and your statement that if there is any need for such information in the future you are available. Males are questioned about their risk of getting someone pregnant as much as females are asked about their risk of pregnancy.

One final note. The sexual history may be that part of the interview in which patients are most likely to ask how you personally feel about something, in this case sexual matters, perhaps because sex is a common experience about which most people have opinions and beliefs. Many people also want to know what is "normal" and discern whether they fit the normal standard. Do not confuse being genuine with giving out personal details of your own life that you are not comfortable discussing. You are not having a conversation with a friend. You are a professional trying to obtain information essential to the diagnosis and management of a patient. Some questions that patients may put to you are clearly inappropriate ("What would you do? Would you have an abortion?" or "Did you have sex before you got married?" or "Don't you think homosexuality is a sin?"), and it is best to answer (no matter what you think) in a polite and straightforward manner, "Well, we're not really here to discuss what I think. I'm more interested in finding out how you feel about this pregnancy" or "about learning that your daughter is gay." In this way, you will help the patient explore his or her own feelings and symptoms as opposed to yours, which are not the focus of the interview.

The Positive ROS

Some patients give a very literal interpretation to the questions in an ROS, answering "yes" to almost every question. When this happens the task seems to become interminably tedious, and the interviewer fears that the history will never end. Sometimes, in addition to being positive, the answers are also given in great detail about relatively trivial matters. For example, while you may want to know if the patient wears glasses, you may have little interest in the fine details of how the patient's refractive error has changed in the past five years or what she feels about her optometrist. A difficult ROS might begin this way:

Dr: Now I'd like to ask you a series of questions just to make sure we haven't missed anything important, okay?

Pt: Fine.

Dr: I'll start with your head and we'll work our way down. Do you get headaches?

Pt: Oh, I'm used to terrific headaches all through my life, and one doctor said it was high blood pressure though I didn't know it at the time.

We seem to be off to a bad start, as we do not expect or desire a severe chronic problem to surface first in the ROS; now, instead of zipping down the list of questions, the interviewer has to stop and ask the details about the headaches. When this happens, usually one of two things is going on: either the physician has failed to inquire in an empathic way about other active problems and significant past medical history or the patient "overinterprets" the question and is describing in great detail a problem that is neither active nor significant.

The best way to deal with this situation is to prevent it in the first place by asking about other active problems and significant past medical problems soon after the questions concerning the present illness. Not only does this maneuver uncover such problems early in the interview but it also facilitates seeing connections between these problems and the present illness. If this technique fails or if you forget to use it, however, there are a number of other approaches. **First,** you may try to bring the patient back to the present with a reminder that the primary interest is those symptoms that are a problem now. **Second,** you may make the questions very general—"Have you ever had any stomach or bowel trouble?"—and ask for further details only when the initial screening is positive. **Third,** you may encourage the patient to filter out the unnecessary details himself by reminding him of the time limitations or asking him to pick out the most important symptoms. **Fourth,** you may undertake the ROS while performing the physical examination and save time in that way.

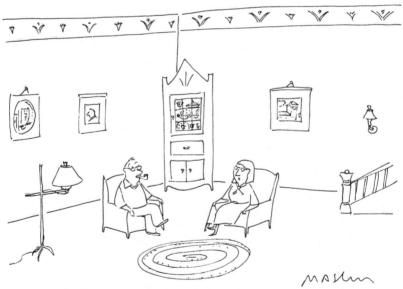

"It's not just my imagination, Carl. Through the use of sophisticated sensing equipment, I've been able to detect a trace of irony in your voice."

Drawing by Maslin; © 1985
The New Yorker Magazine, Inc.

CHAPTER 9

The Difficult Interview, Part 2: Personality Styles and Feeling Problems

When you've once said a thing, that fixes it, and you must take the consequences.

The Red Queen in Lewis Carroll's *Through the Looking Glass*

Another difficulty in medical interviewing arises when the patient's personality style interferes with obtaining objective and precise data. This, of course, is a matter of degree; everyone has a personality style, and under stress, such as that which accompanies illness, distinct coping behaviors identified with certain personalities may become exaggerated. Sometimes identifying a particular style gives you important information: information about how patients perceive their illness, how they "filter" the historic data, and how they generally interact with other people. For example, many patients have a difficult time coping with the hospital schedule and milieu; the hospitalized patient whose nurse did not bring the bedpan promptly and who is generally being treated with a lack of compassion has good reason for fury and may generalize that anger to other personnel, including the medical student or resident who is trying to get a history. The interviewer is confronted with real anger arising out of a real situation, but the anger is not of his or her own making. The best thing to do in this situation is to acknowledge the anger and the patient's right to be angry and to accept the patient's good reasons even if you do not personally agree with them. Allowing the patient time to ventilate his or her feelings in a controlled way permits most interviews to proceed and reinforces your interest in the patient.

Kahana and Bibring (1964) present some useful observations on personality types, which we summarize here, and suggest ways of coping with them during the interview in order to maximize your ability to obtain accurate data. They are (1) the dependent, demanding patient; (2) the orderly, controlled patient; (3) the dramatizing, manipulative patient;

(4) the long-suffering, masochistic patient; (5) the guarded, paranoid patient; and (6) the superior patient. This is a useful classification to orient discussion, though it is unusual to see people who exhibit a truly "pure" style.

The Dependent, Demanding Patient

This type of person strives to impress the physician with the urgent quality of all his or her requests. The patient needs special attention, great reassurance, and constant advice. The doctor first sees an optimistic, compliant "good" patient, but soon finds that the patient expects a limitless amount of attention and care. Groves (1978) described this type of person as one of his "hateful patients" and called him a **dependent clinger.** When the patient's need for "boundless interest and abundant care" is unmet, he or she may become depressed or withdrawn, or blame the doctor in a complaining or vengeful way. The physician who tries to meet every demand risks exhaustion.

In many acutely ill patients dependent tendencies temporarily come to the fore and should be met with active, empathic, and generous care directed toward the patient's physical and emotional comfort. However, when this pattern becomes exaggerated or chronic, the doctor must set limits by stating specific follow-up appointments, specific written instructions, and a clear understanding of the patient's responsibility. It is important for the beginning physician to learn to "protect the patient from promises that cannot be kept and from illusions that are bound to shatter" (Groves, 1978). This is not the patient for whom you should arrange special appointment times, or permit repeated phone calls after hours for nonemergent problems or the repeated calling in to the pharmacy of prescriptions that all seem to run out on different days.

Similarly, within the interview itself, the goal is to set limits for the patient so that the basic task at hand, that of obtaining accurate historic data, can be accomplished. This means that the patient must understand the limits of the "contract" (for example, that you are a student, albeit an interested one, doing a medical history), as well as the need to discuss specific types of information in order for you to understand the patient's problems. Useful techniques include the following:

1. Suspect this problem in new patients who make you feel that you are the only one who has ever cared about them or understood their illness.
2. Avoid making promises that you cannot keep, such as solving a medication or nursing problem.
3. Give the patient responsibility with a statement such as "Perhaps you can talk with the nurses about your pain medication."

4. Remind the patient that your time is limited, despite the fact that you are interested in his or her story. Try a statement such as "You certainly have a lot of important problems, but since my time is so short I'd like to get back to the reason you came into the hospital."
5. Do not take credit for remission in the patient's symptoms, as you will be likely blamed for a relapse, which is sure to follow. Give responsibility to the patient with a statement such as "You're the one who did what was necessary to get better."

The Orderly, Controlled Patient

These patients, when under stress, cope by gaining as much knowledge as possible about their situation, not only to deal with their problem rationally but also to handle their anxiety. These patients are punctual for appointments, conscientious in taking medications, and preoccupied with the right way and the wrong way of carrying out your instructions. Sickness threatens these patients with loss of control. They find the scientific medical approach congenial to their way of thinking and respond well to the professional, systematic sequence of history taking, physical diagnosis, laboratory studies, and therapy. They may present with a list of carefully thought out questions or a precise diary of their symptoms.

Since this type of patient is often on the same "wavelength" as the doctor, it would not appear to present a difficult situation. However, the doctor must be careful to explain the problem thoroughly and describe any laboratory tests or procedures. This is the patient in whom pausing a little longer over auscultation of the heart or inquiring into an area of history seemingly unrelated to the patient's problem may cause excessive anxiety, unless the physician takes care to explain why he or she is doing these things. These patients must be permitted to take charge of their own medical care and be given positive feedback about their efforts and abilities.

Within the interview, this type of patient finds it helpful for the physician to have an orderly and systematic approach, with frequent explanations as to what is happening. Summarizing what you have heard reassures the patient that you are listening and that you are not missing any of the details the patient considers vital to making the diagnosis. This patient will be reassured by your taking notes (he or she does not want you to forget anything important) but alarmed if you suddenly write something down when you have not been writing all along. If the patient asks why you are pursuing a particular line of questioning, make it clear that the purpose is routine or that you want to clarify; do not alarm the patient by revealing the diagnostic hypotheses that may be running around in your head, which led to a particular question. Here is an example:

Dr: How have you been?
Pt: I was trying to remember if I was supposed to call you. I think, I

don't remember when I called last and now I couldn't remember if I was supposed to call you again or not.

Dr: Well, that's fine. I just was hoping that you hadn't tried and not gotten through or something like that. I understand you got new glasses. Has that helped?

Pt: I don't see the slightest difference.

Dr: You're not happy because you're having trouble seeing?

Pt: I'm not happy because I don't see as well as I would like to see. I can't see numbers as well.

Dr: Does the eye doctor give you an explanation?

Pt: Well, he keeps talking. He talks to me referring, speaking to me as "your cataract" and I said to him plainly, I said you referred to my cataract many times. You have never told me I have a cataract. Do I? And he said everyone over 30 years old has a cataract. So that's . . .

Dr: So that's really not an answer. So you don't know whether it's the cataract, whether you have it in both eyes, or whether there's some other problem.

Pt: I don't know, and I can't get a straight answer.

And later in the interview:

Pt: I wanted to tell you about that and I'm trying to think if there is anything else I should tell you. I don't remember anything. Of course, some of the problems are getting worse but I don't consider that something that wasn't expected. I assume that's what we should expect. Everything else is pretty much under control.

Notice how carefully this patient uses her words. When the physician says, "You're having trouble seeing?" she "corrects" this wording with "I don't see as well as I would like to see." She doesn't say that there isn't "anything else I should tell you," she says instead, "I don't remember anything" (and this is interesting, because she is elderly and knows she has a little trouble with her recent memory). Notice her concern with doing the right thing, seeming compliant ("I was trying to remember if I was supposed to call you"). Consider the importance to her of explanations and how disquieted she is by the ophthalmologist's evasiveness ("I can't get a straight answer"). Despite the fact that "some of the problems are getting worse," she tolerates that because "I don't consider that something that wasn't expected." What is good is that "everything else is pretty much under control." Note how the physician is able to clarify her concerns while avoiding explanations about a problem with which he is unfamiliar.

The Dramatizing, Manipulative Patient

This type of patient may first present as interesting and charming, even when he or she dramatizes and makes global statements about symptoms: the pain is "the worst pain I have ever had . . . it's with me all the time, day and night, nothing seems to help . . . I haven't been able to sleep in weeks . . ." This type of person may have a great need to be at stage center and resent the doctor's interest in other duties and other patients. "To the dramatizing, emotionally involved kind of person, a sickness may feel like a personal defect; it means being weak and unattractive, unappreciated, and unsuccessful" (Kahana and Bibring, 1964). These patients are frequently characterized as manipulative and sometimes, particularly when dealing with a doctor of the opposite sex, as seductive. We present some suggestions for interviewing this kind of patient later in this chapter, in the section on manipulative behavior.

The Long-Suffering, Masochistic Patient

Groves (1978) describes this group of patients as "help-rejectors." They give a history of continual suffering from disease, disappointment, and other adversity. They see their lives as a sequence of bad luck. Often they disregard their own needs in order to do things for other people. Despite apparent humility, these patients may have a tendency to be exhibitionistic about their long-suffering fate. With regard to medical care, they feel that no treatment will help; when one symptom goes away, another appears in its place.

The physician must understand that simple reassurance or optimism will not be "bought" by the masochistic patient. He or she will be better able to cooperate in a medical history or a medical treatment if it is seen in the context of adding to his or her "burden," rather than for personal relief. "The physician may have to present the recovery to the patient as a special additional task, if possible for the benefit of others" (Kahana and Bibring, 1964). The doctor might have to share the patient's pessimism, rather than trying to talk it away.

Within the interview, it is important to avoid the minimizing response that is meant to talk the patient out of the severe nature of his suffering. Similarly, it is helpful to avoid overly optimistic or patronizing remarks such as "I'm sure your doctor will have you feeling better in no time." While this patient may not regard talking to a medical student as therapeutic for him or herself, he or she may like the idea of helping you by permitting you to do a history and physical. Accept the patient's pessimism with a statement such as "It sounds as though you don't have much hope of getting better."

Consider the following interchange with an 82-year-old woman who is experiencing failing abilities and is trying to care singlehandedly for her severely demented 89-year-old spouse:

Dr: How have things been going for you?

Pt: Well, not much different. Same as usual. Same problems, same lack of solutions. I'm not saying that anyone would give me a different answer but I still don't have to like it?

Dr: Yeah, you feel that you've gotten that answer to a lot of problems.

Pt: I feel that I've gotten that answer everywhere. Everything that I have problems with. Everything, that is, except Dr. Jackson who wants to operate on my throat . . .

Dr: Which you don't want.

Pt: No. Pretty hopeless, isn't it?

Dr: Well, I think you're doing about as well as anyone could do.

Pt: Well, I don't know, maybe I am. Again I say it's not good enough but I don't suppose there's any good enough in a situation like that.

Dr: How do you feel about the medication right now? Do you think it's helped your spirits at all?

Pt: I like to believe it does. I can't be real sure because I don't know how I'd be feeling without it, but I try to imagine it soothes me some.

Dr: Good.

Pt: I don't think it's doing me any harm.

Dr: Good. What about getting some extra help at home. Have you made any progress with that?

Pt: I don't know. The reason I have resisted is because I had a sister-in-law who could not live alone and she had an endless succession of people that I know stole from her and robbed her.

Dr: The best thing is to get someone that either you or someone that you trust knows well.

Pt: That's true but I don't think that person exists.

Dr: I wish there were something I could do to help.

Pt: I don't expect you to have solutions. It's just how things are. Nothing can change.

This kind of interchange is enough to make any physician feel pretty hopeless as well. Note the patient's repeated return to the theme of no solutions. The most (and it is not much) optimistic she gets is "I like to believe" that the antidepressant she has been taking is helpful, at least "I don't think it's doing me any harm." The physician finally gives up making suggestions and begins to share the patient's pessimism ("I wish there were something

I could do to help"). The patient, in turn, paradoxically reassures the physician ("I don't expect you to have solutions").

The Guarded, Paranoid Patient

These patients are inclined to be suspicious of the doctor and the medical care establishment. They may present a long list of slights from other doctors and openly point out how the illness was mishandled; they will blame others for their illness. During stress, the patient may become "even more fearful, guarded, suspicious, quarrelsome and controlling of others" (Kahana and Bibring, 1964). The doctor may find himself or herself always feeling "on guard" during the interview, as if in some sort of competitive relationship to avoid being "caught."

It is important to give this patient clear explanations of your strategy for diagnosis and treatment. If you are a medical student or house officer, you must pay particular attention to identifying your role and clarifying its limitations. The patient may make provocative statements, but arguing with her or him or ignoring the suspicious attitudes does not help. The best approach is to maintain a friendly and courteous attitude, while acknowledging the patient's beliefs; it is not necessary to agree with these patients, but there is no hope in dissuading them.

Within the interview, a frequent problem you will encounter with these patients is their stated disgust with those caring for them, namely doctors and nurses. The patient may say with great exasperation, "All I want to know is if I've had a heart attack . . . why doesn't my doctor tell me yes or no?" If you were to analyze this request, several issues would have to be resolved: does the doctor know and is not telling, or does he or she simply not know yet and therefore cannot tell? And is there some reason the patient expects to know now as opposed to tomorrow? It is rarely useful to try to unravel such a situation, in part because the answers may not be there and in part because the patient may think that you are taking sides either with or against him or her. It is better to acknowledge and accept the patient's suspicions and frustrations with a statement such as "It must be terribly frustrating, not knowing." Then try to proceed with the history by reminding the patient that, while there is nothing you can do to help with that particular problem, you are interested in hearing more about the symptoms that brought him or her to the hospital.

The Superior Patient

These patients have strong self-confidence and may appear smug, vain, or grandiose. Their behavior in the medical care situation is often that identified by Groves (1978) as the **entitled demander.** They may demand the most senior physician or the most well-known subspecialist and be very condescending or arrogant toward house officers and students. They may attempt to control the physician by making many demands and sometimes by threatening litigation. As Groves (1978) writes, "entitlement serves for some persons the functions that faith and hope serve in better adjusted ones." Often, this patient may react to situations that occur in the hospital with anger and hostility, anger that can impinge on you as the medical student or house officer. Some suggestions for dealing with anger are presented in a subsequent section and are appropriate for this type of patient.

Sometimes a patient makes demands on the physician that he or she would not ordinarily make. Consider this example of a young actor who had never had any difficult interactions with his physician until he developed a "cold or flu or something which normally I would just wait until it went away except I'm involved in a show right now." The dialogue continues:

Pt: And it's the leading role in a rather important production and we open this Thursday *(clears throat)* and I went into this cold.
Dr: You open this coming Thursday.
Pt: And I went into a cold, it feels like it's been in my system for about two weeks, but then on about Thursday it started clearing up, then because of an audition Friday morning I got like six hours of sleep. Friday I started to feel coldish, Saturday I felt terrible, yesterday I felt terrible, so I feel I just need some kind of prescription . . . to be able to deal with it.

So this patient who would "normally just wait" suddenly feels entitled to treatment for a problem that is self-limited and that has no definitive therapy. It is as though the patient is saying, "I know there is no cure for a cold, but since I'm the lead in an important production you must make an exception and cure me." This sounds paradoxic and illogical. In such a situation, the physician might respond:

Dr: There's no cure for the common cold! Actors are no different from anyone else!
Pt: If you won't help me I'll find someone who will.

But things go better if the doctor says:

Dr: I can understand your concern what with this production and all. As you know, there's no cure for the common cold. But why don't I take a look at you and maybe I can recommend something to get the symptoms under control so you'll feel in better form.
Pt: Okay. I sure hope there's something you can do.

PATIENTS WITH SOMATOFORM DISORDERS

You will encounter one group of medical patients whose symptoms are legion but in whom, despite considerable investigation, no good etiology for those symptoms can be identified. These patients have recurrent and multiple physical complaints that span many years, many doctors, many diagnostic work-ups, yet you cannot make any pathophysiologic sense out of the story as a whole. Sometimes the patient will tell you that his or her doctors have "never been able to find anything," but other patients in this group will have been given a sequence of diagnoses and procedures: gallbladder disease followed by cholecystectomy; fibroids followed by hysterectomy; lumbar disc disease followed by a laminectomy; abdominal surgery for lysis of adhesions. Despite these diagnosable disorders to which they ascribe their symptoms, the diseases and the symptoms do not seem to correlate in a way that follows known pathophysiology. Often a procedure is followed by the recurrence of the same or different symptoms. These patients are often identified as "crocks" or "turkeys." Although we question the etiology of their symptoms, their suffering is real.

You must distinguish between the very frequent situation in which (1) physical symptoms are functional or psychophysiologic in origin, based on interactions among life stressors, the autonomic nervous system, and various organ systems that may or may not be diseased; and (2) patients whose somatic complaints represent a primary psychiatric disorder. The former situation includes a large percentage, perhaps the majority, of patients you will see in practice and constitutes an additional portion of suffering for patients with more discrete "organic" diseases, such as anxiety-induced angina pectoris or stress-induced poor control of diabetes. The latter category includes patients who have primary somatoform disorders. Full discussion of these disorders is beyond the scope of this text, but two specific ones must be mentioned because most of the data used in diagnosing them arises from complete and often-repeated medical interviews.

The first is **somatization disorder.** This category defines a group of patients who have chronic but fluctuating physical symptoms that involve several different organ systems, usually beginning during adolescence or early adulthood, and for which no adequate physical explanation can be found. The diagnostic criteria for this disorder, presented in Table 10, are taken directly from the Diagnostic and Statistical Manual of Mental Disorders (DSM-III). You can see that these criteria are quantitative (for example, 12 out of 37 symptoms) and can easily be applied on the basis of a thorough medical history. Often, somatization disorder is confused with another disorder, **hypochondriasis,** the diagnostic criteria for which are presented in Table 11. In hypochondriasis, the patient's problem is "an unrealistic interpretation of physical signs or sensations as abnormal" (DSM-III, p. 249). It is more of a qualitative diagnosis, judging the per-

TABLE 10. Diagnostic Criteria for Somatization Disorder (DSM-III)

A. A history of physical symptoms of several years' duration beginning before the age of 30.

B. Complaints of at least 14 symptoms for women and 12 for men, from the 37 symptoms listed below. To count a symptom as present the individual must report that the symptom caused him or her to take medicine (other than aspirin), alter his or her life pattern, or see a physician. The symptoms, in the judgment of the clinician, are not adequately explained by physical disorder or physical injury, and are not side effects of medication, drugs, or alcohol. The clinician need not be convinced that the symptom was actually present, e.g., that the individual actually vomited throughout her entire pregnancy; report of the symptom by the individual is sufficient.

Sickly. Believes that he or she has been sickly for a good part of his or her life.

Conversion or pseudoneurologic symptoms. Difficulty swallowing, loss of voice, deafness, double vision, blurred vision, blindness, fainting or loss of consciousness, memory loss, seizures or convulsions, trouble walking, paralysis or muscle weakness, urinary retention or difficulty urinating.

Gastrointestinal symptoms. Abdominal pain, nausea, vomiting spells (other than during pregnancy), bloating (gassy), intolerance (e.g., gets sick) of a variety of foods, diarrhea.

Female reproductive symptoms. Judged by the individual as occurring more frequently or severely than in most women: painful menstruation, menstrual irregularity, excessive bleeding, severe vomiting throughout pregnancy or causing hospitalization during pregnancy.

Psychosexual symptoms. For the major part of the individual's life after opportunities for sexual activity: sexual indifference, lack of pleasure during intercourse, pain during intercourse.

Pain. Pain in back, joints, extremities, genital area (other than during intercourse); pain on urination; other pain (other than headaches).

Cardiopulmonary symptoms. Shortness of breath, palpitations, chest pain, dizziness.

TABLE 11. Diagnostic Criteria for Hypochondriasis (DSM-III)

A. The predominant disturbance is an unrealistic interpretation of physical signs or sensations as abnormal, leading to preoccupation with the fear or belief of having a serious disease.

B. Thorough physical evaluation does not support the diagnosis of any physical disorder that can account for the physical signs or sensations or for the individual's unrealistic interpretation of them.

C. The unrealistic fear or belief of having a disease persists despite medical reassurance and causes impairment in social or occupational functioning.

D. Not due to any other mental disorder such as schizophrenia, affective disorder, or somatization disorder.

son's reaction or pattern of reactions over time to ordinary aches and pains or to self-limited illnesses, rather than a sustained pattern of multiple symptoms in multiple organ systems.

These patients are difficult both because your ordinary medical hypotheses do not seem to explain their kind of problem and also because once you have adequately categorized their problem, it is extremely difficult to help them feel better and have less disability. The first step, however, is diagnosis. Thus, you can approach this type of difficult patient by performing a thorough medical interview that gives the relevant data, and by at least considering the hypothesis that a somatoform disorder may be present.

DIFFICULT FEELINGS AND DEFENSES
IN MEDICAL INTERVIEWING

Sometimes the patient's behavior or affect interfere with transmitting adequate information of the kind you need for a precise and accurate history: a patient who feels angry may not wish to speak with you at all; a depressed patient may say too little; a denying patient may be unable to reveal the very symptoms that are so terrifying to him or her. Such situations are likely to make you have several conflicting feelings at once: you may be frustrated at the difficulty in obtaining the history yet feel sorry for the depressed patient; you may be concerned about maintaining a "professional" attitude yet feel defensive or outraged at the angry patient; you may feel pleased at the gratitude shown by the seductive patient yet upset at being manipulated. It is also likely that when you sense strong emotions occurring in the interview you will have some fear about your ability to handle the situation and may, therefore, try to ignore it; or you may feel that it is really not your job as a medical student or a medical doctor to deal with the patient's emotions.

While it may not be your job to manage or treat the cancer patient's depression or the multiple sclerosis patient's denial, it is your job to get an accurate history. When such feelings get in the way of a good history, the feelings will need to be acknowledged in the course of the interview in order for the history to proceed in an efficient and accurate manner. Experienced clinicians find that an empathic response that acknowledges emotional content not only helps the patient feel understood but also actually facilitates the interview, from the point of view of both time (it takes less time) and accuracy (the patient gives better data). While your fear of being overwhelmed by the patient's emotions is a legitimate one, most patients are eager to talk about how they feel and will actually reduce your fear by revealing how they cope with their own personal tragedies.

When feelings interfere with obtaining the history, you should observe carefully the basics of any good interview, which we recapitulate here:

1. Make sure you have the patient's permission to do the interview and that he or she understands the "contract" with you, the student. While this is important to all patients, it is particularly so with the angry patient. Helpful techniques include:

   a. Empathize with the patient's position, stopping short of "accusing" him or her of being angry; you might begin with "I know many doctors have already come in and bothered you . . ."

   b. Elicit the patient's permission, perhaps with a question such as "Is it all right?" If the patient says yes, show your appreciation of his or her cooperation; if the patient says no, accept his or her noncooperation and ask for the patient's reasons in a noncombative way, recognizing his or her right to refuse.

   c. Inform the patient gently of your obligation to do the interview, without attempting to convince or control him or her. Give control to the patient by indicating your willingness to compromise within your limits ("Would it help if I came back in an hour; if I rearranged your pillows; if I talked softer . . . louder, faster . . . slower; if I stood . . . sat").

2. Give the patient **time** to respond, particularly when the subject under discussion is hard for the patient to talk about. Specific techniques include:

   a. Wait for the patient to finish his or her thought or sentence even if he or she hesitates or stumbles over words.

   b. Ask open-ended questions and observe the total communication, including words, gestures, facial expressions, and voice quality.

3. Summarize periodically both the symptom content and the feeling content. Specific uses of summaries include:

   a. To regain control if the patient has wandered off the topic or you are feeling confused. For example, "You are telling me a lot about yourself; let me tell you what I understand so far, because I will want to ask you a specific question."

   b. To prepare the way for a potentially threatening question. For example, "You have had a lot of back pain and from what you tell me, it has also made you quite depressed . . . Has it affected your marriage? Your sex life?"

   c. To clarify and remain "in sync" with the patient, particularly when you notice that the patient feels upset or misunderstood. For example, "Just now as you were describing your pain, you got a very worried look on your face . . . Did I say something that upset you?"

4. Use the interchangeable empathic response to show that you "understand exactly." Try to describe in your own words precisely what the patient's symptoms are, as well as the intensity of emotions being expressed. Look to the patient for confirmation of your statement and acknowledge any corrections. For example:

Dr: So as I understand it you've been having this pain in your chest for the past two to three months and you notice it when you go jogging and you're a little worried about what's causing it *(looks up at patient)*?

Pt: Well, it's not pain exactly, more a discomfort. And actually I'm more than a little worried. My father dropped dead of a heart attack when he was 43 and I'm 42.

Dr: I see, so you're worried that the same thing might happen to you?

Pt: Yeah, I'd really like you to take a cardiogram on me, doc.

5. If you feel lost, acknowledge it as a fact, not as a criticism of the patient; then ask the patient to help you, such as "I'm confused about this, can you help me?" or "I did not quite understand this point, would you help me?"

We now consider patient anxiety, anger, depression, denial, and seductiveness; and in each case, we suggest specific approaches to supplement those we have already discussed.

Anxiety

Every illness produces a mixture of fear and anxiety in the patient. The most common sources of anxiety are feelings of helplessness, fear of dependence, inability to accept warmth or tenderness, and fear of expressing anger. The usual indication that a patient is becoming very anxious is an intensification of his or her customary ways of coping with the world. For example, a compulsive patient will become **more** compulsive; a paranoid patient will become **more** paranoid. The signs of anxiety that you may observe in the interview include facial flushing, sweating, rapid speech, cold hands, fidgeting, or even trembling. The anxious patient may be difficult to interview until the anxiety has been discussed.

All patients are anxious to some extent about their encounter with a physician. Some ways you can help the anxious patient:

1. Be unhurried and calm in your manner.
2. Sympathize, but remember that too much sympathy may magnify the patient's fears.
3. Be very specific as to what you expect of the patient: what cloth-

ing the patient should remove, what position the patient should assume and where.

4. Tell the patient that some anxiety is normal and appropriate: most patients feel this way and it's **okay**.
5. Some patients express their anxiety by asking what you think is causing their symptoms. When this happens it is appropriate to remind the patient that you are a student or that you have not completed your evaluation; in addition you can explore the patient's concerns by asking, "Have you asked your doctor? Why not?" or "What do **you** think is going on?"

Consider this case example. A 57-year-old woman saw her family doctor for an annual examination. She was the sort of person made nervous by doctors and nervous at the thought of a visit even on this day when she had no particular worrisome symptoms. Her red lipstick was coated with antacid as she entered the office; she was so distraught that her stomach felt queezy. It was clear (in retrospect) that just showing up for the exam was a major effort for her. Everything, fortunately, was in order. The physician had only one prescription for her:

Dr: Everything is fine. I have only one recommendation and that is that I'd like you to get a mammogram.
Pt: Oh my God! You mean I've got cancer? Not my breast!
Dr: No, no, of course not. No, I recommend a mammogram for all my patients over the age of 55. It's routine.

And, as though the physician were not leveling with her:

Pt: I couldn't stand to lose a breast, chemotherapy is awful. I already have thinning hair, you know, chemotherapy makes that worse. No, I won't do that, I can't.

In retrospect this patient's fragile adaptation to her encounter with a physician was shattered by one suggestion of a routine test, the purpose of which is to screen for cancer. She seemed to believe that the recommendation was particular, not routine, despite her doctor's protests to the contrary. If we look back at how the doctor introduced the idea, we notice what may have seemed to the patient a contradiction: "everything's fine . . . get a mammogram." This anxiety-ridden patient thinks, "if everything's fine, why do I need a mammogram?" The physician may have been able to achieve his aim (that of her getting a mammogram which, by the way, she never agreed to) by saying:

Dr: Everything's fine. Your exam is completely normal. Just like you come for a Pap test because you know that's routine in all

> women, so we now routinely recommend a mammogram for all women your age. Do you know what that is? Have you ever had one done?

In this instance, the physician is more reassuring because he is specific about what is "fine" ("your exam is completely normal"), he frames the "routine" nature of the mammogram in a concrete way to which the patient can relate, just as she has come for a "routine" Pap test, and he anticipates the patient's worry by explaining the reason for the test **before** the patient can spin a fantasy of calamity.

Anger

While anxiety may facilitate our feeling sympathetic toward the patient, many physicians find anger more difficult to handle. Patients may behave in a hostile manner for many different reasons. Most of the time the reasons have nothing to do with you personally; rather, they relate to the patient's situation, such as inconsiderate care by hospital staff, failure of the patient's physician to communicate, or the patient's unique response to his or her illness, disability, or prognosis. What makes one patient depressed may make another patient angry. Some ways to handle anger include:

1. Recognize and acknowledge anger with a statement such as "I can see/hear/feel you are angry, frustrated" or "Waiting so long made you angry." If you are not sure that what you are hearing is anger, ask: "Are you feeling angry?"
2. Accept the anger by continuing to **listen to the patient** while explaining the situation in a neutral fashion, even though a logical explanation will not necessarily change the patient's feelings. Do not take sides.
3. Explore the contributing factors and identify the underlying feelings such as fear, hurt, disappointment, powerlessness. Accept the patient's reason even if you do not personally agree with it. Remember, **there is always a reason**, although it may not be immediately evident.
4. If the patient's anger is justifiably directed at you, acknowledge your mistake. You are learning; mistakes are unavoidable; you can learn from them and correct them. If the patient's anger is not related to you, help the patient recognize ways he can deal with the anger-provoking situations. For example:

> Pt: You're just as insensitive as the rest of 'em.
> Dr: I guess that was a foolish question to ask. Now that I understand you a little better, do you think we could start over?

This next patient regretted being interviewed in front of a group of residents at a psychiatric case conference. She is talking to her physician following the conference:

> Pt: I now know what it's like to be poor. I never would have been at that conference if I had my own private doctor. I know what it's like to be a guinea pig. That doctor asked about my early childhood when what I needed was someone to find out what's been going on over the last ten years and how tough life has been for me so that he could help me. I thought he would be able to give me something to help my nerves right now, not just talk about my grandmother.

While this patient reminds us of the entitled demander and indeed may be one, she is clear, if we listen, as to what is so upsetting to her. She is focused on how she feels at present and is looking for relief from feelings that are unpleasant. Talking about what seemed to her to be ancient history confused and frustrated her. The conference ended apparently without a prescription or clear plan of action, and although the physician was trying to remedy the situation, the patient may not have known that. Here an explanation and an acknowledgment of her feelings are in order:

> Dr: It certainly must seem strange to talk about old things when you feel so bad now and want relief. I can certainly understand your frustration. Actually the reason I wanted to talk with you is to discuss what to do next to get you to feel better. Because Dr. Smith had some good ideas which I think we should try. In fact, he suggested some medication which he thinks will be helpful and I think so too.

The other aspect of her anger was a sense of being on display or of being experimented with (perhaps two sides of the same coin). She may have been unaware of the conference format, requiring her to sit in front of a room full of strange doctors whom she had never met before. If she was not prepared for what was to occur, as she should have been by someone, her physician can only apologize:

> Dr: I'm sorry, I guess I didn't really explain what was supposed to happen very well to you. I'm sorry you felt uncomfortable. But I did learn a lot about you which I think will help me to take better care of you.
> Pt: Okay. What I really need is to feel better.

Depression

Depression may be a manifestation of a diagnosable psychiatric disorder, a response to recent tragedy (such as death of a spouse), an expression of a chronic approach to life in general (the pessimist), or a more transient feeling state. Depression may be the underlying problem in a substantial proportion of those patients who consult their physicians with complaints of fatigue, weakness, lack of energy, insomnia, backache, or headache, but depression as a **response to illness** is equally common. Depressive characteristics include feelings of worthlessness, hopelessness, apathy, and guilt, together with a profoundly empty and lonely feeling. These are manifest in the patient's manner, tone of voice, posture, and speech; thinking is slow, speech sparse, and voice volume low. The patient may speak softly, looking down or away from you and may be tearful. Sometimes a statement such as "You look sad" gives the patient an opportunity to talk about depressed feelings and thereby facilitates other more "medical" aspects of the history.

Some patients have endured such tragic events that you yourself fear being overwhelmed with the sadness of it all. In such instances, it is appropriate to say that you, too, find the situation sad; in this way you make it clear to the patient that you are a fellow human being with feelings. However, in addition to this commonality you are also a professional, and your feelings should be used in a constructive way to help the patient. Here is an example that has both a feeling focus and a constructive focus. The patient is a 57-year-old woman, who had coronary bypass surgery at the age of 53, followed two years later by a left radical mastectomy for aggressive carcinoma of the breast, who is now suffering from metastatic disease, and who is about to lose her health insurance coverage because her husband's business is failing and they can no longer afford it.

> Dr: Gee, a lot of bad things have happened to you. You must be a pretty strong person to have endured all this . . . How have you managed?
>
> Pt: Well, I have my faith . . . and my family has been just wonderful to me.

Notice how the physician acknowledges the feeling content but, instead of getting deep into the tragedy, allows the patient to express her strength and her coping style. This technique serves the dual purpose of keeping both patient and physician from being overwhelmed.

Some useful questions to assess the depth of depression, including assessment of suicide risk, are:

Do you get pretty discouraged (or blue)?

What do you see for yourself in the future? How do you see the future?

Do you ever feel that life isn't worth living? Or that you'd just as soon be dead? Or that you just can't go on?

And, if answers to the above questions so indicate, you should pursue the question of suicide:

Have you ever thought of doing away with yourself? Ending your life? Of suicide?

Did you ever think about how you would do it?

What would happen to your family (parents, spouse, and so on) after you were dead?

It is important to give the patient time to answer these questions. Most patients are relieved to talk about feelings of suicide; such discussion does not put the idea of suicide into their heads. Often the best follow-up questions are simply statements such as "Tell me more about these feelings" or "Tell me more about it" or the use of simple prompters and facilitators such as "Mm hmm," followed by silence to allow the patient to continue. Often this technique uncovers information vital to the diagnostic process:

Dr: You look sad. Is it about this chest pain you're having or something else?

Pt: I guess I am sad. My chest has been hurting all week. Well . . . see . . . I don't know if I can say it . . . I get all choked up . . . excuse me (trying to hold back tears). My mother died on Monday. Every time I think about her I get this choked up feeling in here and it starts to hurt like my angina down into my arm.

Here the physician discovers the crucial connection between an exacerbation of her patient's angina and the recent death of the patient's mother.

Denial

Denial is a common response to illness that most patients have, at least to some degree. It is the feeling that "this isn't really happening to me" or "I can't believe it" or "that wasn't blood I saw in my bowel movement—at least, I don't think it was." In some patients the denial is strong enough that they either ignore or do not remember symptoms, or they may play down a worrisome symptom and report it as a trivial event: "I had a little pain in my chest but it only lasted an hour." Only later do you find out that the pain was not only severe but associated with nausea and sweating and a feeling of impending doom. While some patients play down the symptoms themselves, others deny the emotional impact of a particular diagnosis or prognosis. At times, it is hard to tell the difference between optimism and denial; for example, the patient with a potentially lethal disease who smiles and says "I know I can beat it." When patients accept bad news with apparent equanimity, it is difficult to know whether they are "handling it well" or denying some or all of the meaning of the diagnosis or prognosis. While denial can lead to serious delays in seeking care, it is also a useful mechanism by which many patients cope with bad news. The clinician, therefore, should handle denial with circumspection and respect, while trying to assess the patient's understanding of what is happening. Some useful techniques include:

1. Accept denial as the patient's unique and current experience.
2. Inform him gently and calmly that many people feel differently, including you: "Most people feel very sad when they hear they have a serious illness" or "I guess I would be worried."
3. Drop the subject if the patient is silent. He may come back to it, tentatively saying that once or twice he has felt as you described.

Consider this example of a young woman who came to the doctor for a "check-up." This was her first visit to this physician. On palpating the abdomen, the physician found a large mass which, on pelvic examination and subsequent ultrasound proved to be an enormous uterine fibroid. The patient seemed unaware of its presence, despite the fact that the mass was the size of a five-month pregnancy. When she was told that a hysterectomy might be necessary, she seemed unconcerned. The physician needed to find out if this 30-year-old woman who had not yet had children understood what a hysterectomy would mean to her and was accepting that, or simply did not understand the implications of the surgery. (The physician's concern was, perhaps, heightened by the fact that the patient seemed to have denied the presence of a large abdominal mass.)

Dr: You don't seem very concerned at the idea of a hysterectomy.
Pt: Well, if I have to have it, that's it.
Dr: Do you know what a hysterectomy is?
Pt: Well, I guess that's when they take everything out.
Dr: Well, actually, it means removal of the uterus or womb, that's where this fibroid is. Now this tumor is an overgrowth in the muscle, but even though it's not cancer, it may be impossible to remove without removing the uterus. Now your ovaries, which are the glands next to the uterus that make female hormones like estrogen—you've heard of estrogen?—okay, the ovaries would

not be removed. *(Draws picture)* They would stay, so your hormones would still work right.

Pt: But I still couldn't have babies.

Dr: That's right, you couldn't have babies. What do you think about that?

Pt: I don't know. I guess I never thought much about it, not being married and all, but I guess it hasn't really hit me yet. I'm more worried about the operation itself.

Notice how the physician gently probes the patient's knowledge and offers a clear explanation as to what will happen. The patient is not denying the outcome of the surgery but is, perhaps, delaying dealing with it pending resolution of her more immediate fears about the operation itself.

Manipulative and Seductive Behavior

We have emphasized the importance of allowing the patient to tell her story in her own words with some direction from the interviewer but without the high control style that produces poor data. However, there are times when the issue of control is central to the interview process; the patient wants too much control, and you are unable to obtain the information you need. Sometimes the problem permeates the entire history. At other times, the problem is limited to a particular part of the history, for example, the patient with a drug problem who steers the discussion into other areas every time you approach the question of substance abuse.

Sometimes the patient wants to control you and engages in a type of behavior not usually appropriate to a professional relationship, such as noticing your new watch or hairstyle, or complimenting you on your good taste, or asking you personal questions about your social relationships or your sexual preference or whether you have ever had an abortion. Here are some guidelines for dealing with this type of behavior in the interview:

1. Listen and observe the patient as he or she demonstrates this type of behavior. Think: What does the patient gain by this behavior?
2. Control the urge to engage in open warfare for control of the interview by feeding back what you hear and clarifying points.
3. Remain calm, gentle, and firm, using frequent summaries to regain or stay in control.
4. Remain descriptive, not judgmental or evaluative; focus on the how, not the why. For example, "I've noticed that when I try to ask you about drug use you tend to change the subject," **not** "Why don't you answer my question?"
5. Identify the strengths of the patient and feed them back by establishing a profile of the premorbid person, as well as of the patient you are currently interviewing.

6. Remember that if the patient with chronic pain has been suffering for months, or years, he or she will survive suffering one more minute, hour, day, week, month.

7. If the patient asks you a personal question or one you are uncomfortable about answering, try reflecting back to the patient with a statement such as "Well, we're really not here to talk about my opinion . . . I'm interested in hearing more about you. How did **you** handle that?"

8. Reframe seductive behavior positively as one of the patient's many possible moves toward attaining goals in his or her life, such as "I see that you enjoy being an attractive person and you enjoy being with a man and being noticed by him and taken care of by him. How do you meet those needs in your life?" or "So you are a widower; how has that been for you?"

A thorough history in a respectful atmosphere where you demonstrate you are in charge is the best way to build a solid relationship with the patient and to establish a treatment plan that will be acceptable.

PATIENTS' AND PHYSICIANS' FEELINGS ABOUT EACH OTHER

The interaction between physician and patient may be highly charged with emotion. This relationship may bring out attitudes and behaviors reflecting previous relationships that either patient or doctor have had. The sicker the patient, the more helpless and dependent he or she is, the more likely it is that his or her attitude toward the doctor will reflect a great deal of previously learned attitudes and experiences. Sometimes these attitudes are manifest in ways that appear totally irrational to the interviewer. For example, a patient who has had an angry competitive relationship with his father, perceiving the male physician as a powerful authority, may become antagonistic, sarcastic, and competitive even though the physician has done nothing that would ordinarily elicit such a response; female physicians may encounter irrational responses based on the patient's early experiences with being mothered. Although you may not be able to figure it out at the time, there is always a reason for what looks like irrational behavior. You can only maintain a respectful attitude toward the patient and use the techniques outlined above to establish rapport and obtain the history.

Your interaction with the patient is, of course, two-sided; thus, while patients have feelings about you, you will most certainly have feelings about your patients. You may try to hide them or even wonder if it is appropriate to have such feelings. You will like some patients a lot, and others less so; there may be some that you actively dislike. Some will make you angry; others you will dread. Some will make you laugh, and you will wonder whether it is "professional" to do so. You may even feel "attracted" to certain patients of the opposite sex and feel embarrassed or behave awkwardly. The best approach to such feelings is first to identify and acknowledge them, at least to yourself. Think: How is the patient making me uncomfortable? And why? The answer to the "how" questions will allow you to identify behaviors in the patient that are helpful in your assessment. For example, ask yourself, "Do I dread seeing this patient because he makes too many demands on me?" If so, he may be the "entitled demander" we spoke of earlier and require particular attention to your interviewing technique. Or perhaps you feel uncomfortable with another patient because she's depressed, or because she's dying and you are afraid that there is nothing you can do for her. Remember, this is your problem, not the patient's. You may want to share such feelings with helpful colleagues, and, finally, as you gain considerable comfort with these feelings, you will be able to share them with the patient and so improve his or her self-understanding. The opportunity to create a real connection with your patient can be the basis for a professional intimacy as you learn more about each other over time.

CHAPTER 10

Compliance and Negotiation in the Clinical Interview

> The free practitioner . . . treats their diseases by going into things thoroughly from the beginning in a scientific way, and takes the patient and his family into confidence. Thus he learns something from the sufferers, and at the same time instructs the invalid to the best of his powers. He does not give his prescriptions until he has won the patient's support, and when he has done so, he steadily aims at producing complete restoration of health by persuading the sufferer into compliance.
>
> Plato, *The Laws*

Most treatment in medicine includes a **behavioral component** or **vector**; the patient must do something, and how you interact with the patient is likely to influence whether or not the patient takes his or her medication or follows other advice you give. Comatose patients in the hospital receive their intravenous fluids and medications with little if any compliance necessary on their part, but it is difficult to imagine other medical care situations in which the behavioral vector is not significant. Although "compliance" is a common term in medical parlance, it has several drawbacks: (1) it suggests that the physician's orders are uniquely right and that any patient failure to be 100 percent compliant must mean that the outcome will be less than successful; and (2) it suggests a passive, "plastic" patient rather than an active, participating one. The word "adherence" escapes from the second connotation to some extent, but it still contains the first. The patient must adhere, albeit actively, to the doctor's correct regimen. We prefer to talk simply about the patient's behavior with regard to treatment and instructions and to consider how much the physician himself or herself influences that behavior. In this way we describe the behavioral vector present in any doctor-patient interaction.

Dozens of studies have shown that patient "compliance" with medications, particularly over the long term, averages around 50 percent (Sackett and Haynes, 1976). This figure considered by itself is not very informative, because it does not tell us whether 50 percent of the patients comply 100 percent of the time with their treatment, while the others stop taking it entirely; or whether 100 percent of the people actually take their medications about half the time; or which subgroups among them are more or less likely to be more or less compliant. The 50 percent figure also need not bear any direct relationship to the success of therapy. It could well be that a medication is effective when taken in lower doses or less frequently than prescribed, even though it may be more efficacious were it actually taken in the prescribed manner. On the other hand, lest we forget the negative side of our therapies, patients would be more likely to have side effects and to develop toxic reactions if they all took every medication prescribed in full dosage. Although complete adherence to all prescribed drugs would probably lead to somewhat better outcomes with regard to the original illnesses, it would surely also lead to more iatrogenic illness.

In reality, however, your treatment of the patient is not just the drug you prescribe. A prescription is but a small part of the complete interaction you have with the patient, an interaction that has focal, behavioral, and symbolic influences on that person and his or her illness. Even as you complete your initial interview, your history and physical examination, you must begin to bring these other influences to bear in your management of the patient. You may simply be ordering further diagnostic studies, while explaining your preliminary findings and expecting the patient to return to see you again. Even so, you want to do whatever you can to make sure that the patient actually obtains the studies, follows your advice, and returns to your office. You also want to do what you can to make the patient feel better starting today, rather than next week or next month. You want in some way, if possible, to reduce the patient's anxiety and to relieve his or her suffering. This chapter deals with the behavioral vector, or how you influence the patient's attitudes and behaviors through transmitting clear information, understanding what the patient believes and expects, and negotiating a plan of action. These activities reduce anxiety, an issue we will discuss more in the next chapter.

The skills involved in facilitating the behavioral healing vector can be grouped under three headings: (1) the **cognitive** sphere, dealing with the actual transmittal, understanding, and retention of information; (2) the **meaning** sphere, dealing with the patient's beliefs about himself, his illness, and what can or should be done about it; and (3) the **negotiation** sphere, dealing with the process through which the physician uses his or her knowledge about the patient's personality, psychodynamics, beliefs, and values to achieve a "best-negotiated" behavioral outcome.

THE COGNITIVE SPHERE

Why don't patients always follow their doctor's instructions? Ley (1976) suggested four hypotheses to explain noncompliant behavior: (1) the personality hypothesis, which holds that something in the patient's basic personality structure interferes; (2) the psychodynamic hypothesis, which holds that some important defense mechanism, such as denial, prevents compliance; (3) the interpersonal hypothesis, in which affective problems arising from the doctor-patient interaction prevent full compliance; and (4) the cognitive hypothesis, which holds that the problem has to do with communication per se—words and concepts—and the simple recall of what the doctor said. While each of these must play a part at least some of the time, Ley (1976) favors the cognitive explanation and has demonstrated through his many studies that patients do not remember a good deal of what the doctor tells them, and they cannot do what the doctor recommends if they fail to remember what medication to take or how to take it.

The first step in "compliance," conceptually at least, is that the patient understands what the doctor is saying and remembers it. Investigators agree that patients on the average remember 50 to 60 percent of the information doctors give them immediately thereafter, and about 45 to 55 percent several weeks later (Joyce and co-workers, 1969; Ley, 1978). Interestingly, neither the intelligence nor age of the patient seem to be important factors in how much is remembered. Others have found that writing down the information, which on the surface would appear to be a fail-safe method, does not, in fact, necessarily lead to a better outcome in terms of better compliance or more information remembered. Of note, patients who have a moderate level of anxiety about their problem are more likely to remember what the doctor tells them than if they have either very high (paralyzing and distracting) or very low (nonmotivating) anxiety levels.

It is clear that patients will be more satisfied with their care and will follow instructions better if they remember what the doctor tells them. Here is an example of the final part of a diagnostic interview in which, among other problems, the doctor appears to pay little attention to the cognitive sphere in his communication:

> Dr: Okay, well Mr. H., you've been having ah, these problems for some time and ah, I think they warrant ah, further investigation. I'm not quite sure right now, some of your symptoms ah, seem to be upper GI but some seem to be ah, colonic as well. It could be an ulcer problem, it could be inflammatory bowel disease. I think the first thing to do is to schedule a proctoscopy and then we'll go on from there. I can do the procto in the office here

later on this week—the nurse can give you an exact time—and meanwhile ah, we'll get you scheduled for the ah, x-rays. You'll need a barium enema, probably air contrast, and then an upper GI series . . .

Pt: Is that test you mentioned, is that where you insert a tube in my rectum? I had one of those about two years ago, I could hardly stand it . . .

Dr: Well, it's not the most comfortable thing, but it is important, it's the only way you can get the rectum—look at it, see the problem. It's not as bad as you think . . .

Pt: The main problem I'm having is this bloated feeling, and the indigestion. I didn't think it was so serious. Isn't there some medicine?

Dr: As you said, it's been bothering you for quite some time so I think we ought to get to the bottom of it. You can never be too careful. The problem with the GI tract is that, a lot of times, symptoms seem to blend together and it's hard to know what your dealing with unless you look.

Pt: Do you think it might be something serious, I mean like an ulcer or something . . .

Dr: Well, it could be an ulcer, but it's not typical. I think we'll just have to do the work-up and see. In the meantime, I'm going to give you an antispasmotic drug to take, you can take it with every meal and at bedtime. I'll give you a prescription. We'll see what happens.

Let us focus first on the doctor's initial statement in this interview segment. How might this doctor have presented the information in such a way as to facilitate understanding? **First,** he could have used words and phrases more likely to be understood by the patient. The phrase "inflammatory bowel disease" and the term "proctoscopy" should not be employed unless the doctor intends to explain them, or at least check back with the patient to determine whether he knows what they mean. Medical jargon can creep into any conversation. It is almost as if English becomes the doctor's second language and he or she must mentally translate each concept from "medicalese." You will find that some concepts (as opposed to descriptive words like "proctoscopy") are difficult to explain, but anything important to the patient that goes on in his or her body **can** be described in plain language. Often, a difficulty in translation results from our own failure to have fully mastered a particular concept.

Second, the doctor in the example could have been concrete and specific about what problems he was considering that he had ruled out, what the steps in diagnosis would entail, and why they are important. On the contrary, the doctor spoke in abstract and general terms like "further investigation" and "go on from there." What does that mean? We understand that he is uncertain of the actual diagnosis, but he has failed to categorize explicitly just what the options are and, more importantly for the patient at that point, what the likely outcome will be: Will I get better? Will I probably need surgery? Is it serious? Eric Cassell refers to this failure to be explicit by calling it **vague reference**, a technique in communicating with patients that often leads to increased anxiety about the problem (Cassell, 1979), because it leaves the patient room to imagine "the worst."

Third, this doctor could have stated the most important information concisely at the beginning. Patients are more likely to remember the initial chunks of information presented than they are to recall information presented later in a discussion. You should "hook" the patient's memory by giving a succinct statement that puts the problem in a frame of reference and leads to "here's how we'll deal with it." The doctor could then employ another technique, **repetition,** to bring home the salient points during his subsequent discussion with the patient.

Fourth, at the end of the segment, the doctor could have inquired about how much the patient understood and given him some feedback about that understanding. He could have encouraged questions. The simple technique of requesting the patient to repeat what you have said, and then giving feedback, substantially increases patient satisfaction and also increases accurate recall of information (Bertakis, 1977).

Taking the example as a whole, notice that the doctor is sharing his uncertainty with the patient. The clinical situation is truly ambiguous, and the doctor's statements accurately convey that fact. However, the **manner** in which the doctor deals with this ambiguity appears neither to be educational nor to relieve the patient's anxiety. It creates new questions, and leaves the old one ("Is it something serious?") unanswered. Moreover, the doctor has really communicated no specific information or advice to the patient about his problem. While the diagnosis is admittedly still unclear, the doctor **does** have a good deal more knowledge about what the symptoms mean and what might be done about them than the patient has. Even though he himself is uncertain, the doctor could use this opportunity to decrease some of the uncertainty that the patient suffers from, while mobilizing the patient's efforts to address the problem constructively.

In summary, communication need not be vague or confusing even if the situation is uncertain. Here is an example of how the same doctor might, on a better day, share his findings and arrive at a plan with the patient:

Dr: Well, Mr. H., you've had a difficult time with this problem but I believe we'll be able to get to the bottom of it and find out what's wrong. We will have to do some additional tests, though, before we can say for sure. Your main symptoms, the cramps you get and the loose bowels, are most likely caused by a problem in your colon, one that we call irritable bowel syndrome. That means that there's a spasm in the muscles of your large bowel and that gives you the cramps and so on. But your other symptoms, that bloated feeling in the stomach and pain up there, they also suggest an acid problem, like ulcer or gastritis.

Pt: Are any of those serious?

Dr: They're all medical problems that can be treated or cured. There's nothing to suggest that you have something really serious like cancer, for example. It could be an ulcer, but I think it's more likely that irritable bowel syndrome can explain all of your symptoms.

Pt: I really want to get to the bottom of this, I just can't take it anymore. I just can't get my work done feeling like I do now.

Dr: It sounds like these attacks have really gotten to you . . .

Pt: I'd say I'm almost paralyzed.

Dr: Okay, I understand. What I'd like to do is to schedule some tests today. One of them is a proctoscopy, that's a procedure in which I insert a tube into your rectum. I can look through it and check the lining of your bowel, like for irritation or hemorrhoids. You'll come back to my office for that. The other two tests are x-rays, one of the large bowel and one of the stomach and small bowel . . .

Pt: Do you think it might be something serious, like an ulcer or something?

Dr: What are you thinking about? Possibly it could be an ulcer . . .

Pt: Well, ulcers can kill you, can't they?

Dr: It sounds like you heard something bad about ulcers.

Pt: My uncle bled to death from one. First they said it was an ulcer, then it didn't heal, he couldn't eat anything, finally they found out it was cancer.

Dr: And you're worried that this could be cancer, even if the tests show something else?

Pt: I don't know. Like I say, I can't take it anymore. My nerves are part of it, maybe.

Dr: Let's take this a step at a time. First, your symptoms and my examination do not show any suggestion of cancer; we have no reason to suspect it. As I said, it really sounds like either an acid problem or irritable bowel, that's the most likely. Let me explain that a little more . . .

This time the doctor has done a number of things to influence the patient to have the diagnostic studies and take the medication as directed. The patient may well be more satisfied than in our first example and go home less anxious about his condition. **Several of the techniques the doctor**

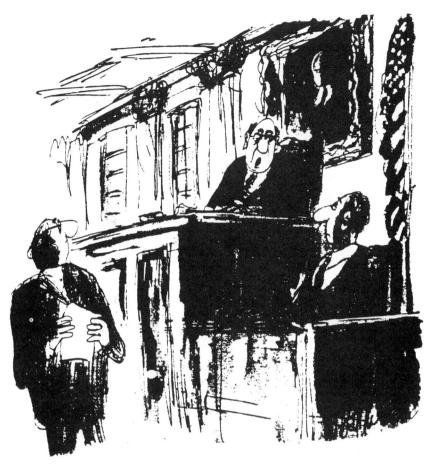

"If the answer is no, <u>say</u> 'No.' Don't say 'Not really.'"

Drawing by Joe Mirachi: © 1984
The New Yorker Magazine, Inc.

used were in the cognitive sphere—they ensured better transfer of information. These are summarized in Table 12. The doctor also actively elicited and then listened to what the patient believed ("my uncle bled to
death . . .") and took that into account. In other words, he also addressed
the conceptual and affective meaning sphere.

TABLE 12. Maximizing Recall of Information: The Cognitive Sphere

1. Use plain English, rather than medical jargon.
2. Use concrete and specific language, rather than vague reference.
3. State the important message first, then use repetition to reinforce it.
4. Ask the patient to restate the message, and give corrective feedback.

THE MEANING SPHERE: CONCEPTUAL AND AFFECTIVE

Consider the following excerpt from a conversation between a doctor and a patient who has sought medical care because of epigastric pain and "heartburn."

> Pt: I take shots for allergies and I take two aspirins every day for my blood pressure . . . I don't eat any sugar, any salt.
> Dr: Two aspirins for . . .
> Pt: Every morning.
> Dr: For that, why do you take that?
> Pt: Trying, trying to thin out my blood to keep my pressure down, I try to keep it around 100.
> Dr: I see.

Later in the same interview the patient comes back to the issue of aspirin and blood pressure in this way:

> Pt: But I always take two aspirins, I've taken two aspirins for years.
> Dr: Where did you get into that habit?
> Pt: Ah, when I was in the military in '68 and '69.
> Dr: Um hmm.
> Pt: German doctor told me that ah, if you take two aspirins with milk in the morning he says, it lowers your blood pressure and thins things out.
> Dr: Um hmm.
> Pt: And I've always, my blood pressure is always like 100, 110, its real low.

This person **has** a perfectly logical belief regarding aspirin and blood pressure if you accept his basic premise. He assumes that high blood pressure is caused by "thick" blood. If so, and if aspirin thins the blood, it is reasonable to take aspirin to prevent hypertension. This particular belief is likely to be a simple piece of misinformation. It could easily be remedied by the doctor explaining that blood pressure and blood coagulation involve two entirely different physiologic systems. It would be particularly important to address this issue if the patient were indeed found to be hypertensive and treatment recommended, or if he had peptic ulcer disease and could not take aspirin.

This piece of "folk physiology" is reminiscent of the "high blood/low blood" beliefs among many American blacks and southern whites (Snow, 1974). These groups confuse high blood pressure with "high blood" or excessive blood volume, which is thought to cause strokes when the excess blood backs up into the brain. Anemia means "low blood" to them; too little blood puts a strain on the person's heart. It is difficult for patients with this understanding of physiology to accept the notion that they have hypertension and anemia at the same time. It just does not make sense for them to have both high and low blood. Physicians who treat Hispanic patients may encounter similar problems in prescribing a "hot" medicine for a "hot" disease. Many Puerto Ricans and Mexican-Americans subscribe to a traditional folk physiology that requires a balance of "humors" for health. Illness is believed to be an imbalance between the "hot" and "cold." Certain diseases are characterized as being "cold" and others as being "hot." Medicines and other treatments are also divided in this way. You treat a "cold" illness with a "hot" medicine, to restore balance. The unsuspecting physician who prescribes hot-for-hot may well have a reluctant and noncompliant patient (Harwood, 1971).

Often physicians can accept the health and healing beliefs of people belonging to other cultures, but they frequently fail to take into account the wide spectrum of folk physiology and healing practices presented by most ordinary people in our society, regardless of age, cultural background, or education. People everywhere are concerned about the origin of their symptoms and the outcome of their illnesses, and so they formulate hypotheses about them. They learn from experience, from books, from television, and from friends. They often seek help from a variety of sources. Sick people do not usually read medical textbooks, nor do they have the same blind faith in scientific medicine that medical students and physicians often have. When you are sick it is difficult to believe that the illness is a random event, a matter of probability: 22 percent of persons exposed to this virus become clinically ill, and of these, 14 percent develop jaundice. But why me? Why did I get hepatitis? Illness is not value-free or meaning-free. We live in a world of symbols and interpretation. We personalize events.

The person who visits a doctor comes with some beliefs about the illness. Part of these may be conceptual or intellectual: What is the cause? How serious is it? What treatment do I need? The beliefs may be specific to this one episode ("I was in a draught," or "I stayed up all night to study for my Serbo-Croatian final"); or more general notions about human disease ("Disease comes from vitamin deficiencies," or "A lot of illness comes from spinal problems"). Another part of the patient's beliefs is affective or personal. Particularly if it is serious or chronic illness, your patient will have wondered, "What does this mean to me? Is it a punishment? Is it a challenge? Will I die like Uncle Harry whose cancer started the same way?"

Although everyone who is even a little sick has some such conceptual and personal meanings for his or her suffering, we do not always ask about them explicitly in the medical history nor discuss them as we plan further tests or treatment. If the patient did not have some faith in medicine, he or she would not be in the emergency room or your office. If you are empathic and demonstrate your competence, the patient will have even more faith in you personally. You will help change the meaning of his or her illness by simply doing a good job. However, in certain situations, belief factors appear to play a more significant role, and you will not be able to help the patient optimally or influence his or her behavior until you understand and deal with them.

How can you tell if you are dealing with a situation in which belief factors are influencing the patient's behavior or the disease outcome? **One clue** is in acute illness when the disease gets better with therapy, but the sickness seems to persist; or when you successfully treat symptoms, and new symptoms keep appearing when the old ones disappear. You might learn this on an initial interview if your patient tells you that ever since his bout of pneumonia two months ago, he has not had any energy and has developed insomnia.

A **second clue** is in chronic illness when the condition is always poorly controlled despite your attempts to prescribe usually effective drugs. You suspect the patient is noncompliant but cannot prove it and do not know why. Often, you become angry with these people who do not seem to understand simple English ("I told her time and again, and explained the pills over and over") or appear to be unconcerned or, worse, self-destructive.

A **third "red flag"** arises when your patient's suffering and disability are far in excess of the evident disease. A patient might bring in a disability form for you to complete because she has "high blood pressure and arthritis." Her blood pressure is mildly elevated but that, of course, is asymptomatic. She has some Heberden's nodes (degenerative osteophytes at the distal interphalangeal joints) but these are usually asymptomatic. She sometimes has aching in her shoulder, but the x-ray films are normal. Yet the patient believes she is disabled. She may well be, but you must address the meaning of her problems to find out why.

A **fourth and particularly problematic clue** is an extension of the third: chronic sickliness and disability without any identifiable disease. A prime example of this is "culture-bound illness," a phrase anthropologists use to describe characteristic illnesses that originate from and are sustained entirely by sociocultural factors. One such syndrome that occurs among Latin American people is "susto," or magical fright. A young woman may, for example, develop this illness shortly after she marries, enters her husband's family system, leaves her own family, and assumes new responsibilities with little support; she may become weak, dizzy, lose her appetite, and suffer from other characteristic symptoms that indicate that she is "a sustado" (Uzzell, 1978). Such a sickness is best treated by a traditional healer, a curandero, rather than by a medical doctor. This is not an imaginary problem; it can be quite malignant. The physiologic changes are real and uncontrolled, even if they have psychosocial origins. The "ghost sickness," suffered by American Plains Indians, and "neurasthenia," a common European and American ailment around the turn of the 20th century, are other examples of culture-bound illness. We are likely to have such culture-bound problems in our culture, but they may not be as clearly visible to us as such. It is certain, however, that you will encounter many patients who are sorely disabled, who suffer greatly, and in whom you can discover no disease.

Table 13 presents questions that will help you make an assessment of patient beliefs as part of your complete interview. They constitute a kind of screening test to ascertain whether your patient's beliefs and expectations fall within a "normal" range, a range in which they will not seriously conflict with medical explanations or treatment; or whether they fall outside this range, in which case they might prevent you from effectively influencing behavior. We have adapted these questions from Kleinman, Eisenberg, and Good (1978) and arranged them to indicate three types of meaning each illness can have: **descriptive, conceptual, and affective or personal.**

The first, descriptive, level simply recaps what we discussed in Chapter 3. You must find out what your patient identifies as the problem for which he or she is seeking help. The "ostensible reason for coming" or chief complaint may not, in fact, be the "actual reason for coming" (Bass and Cohen, 1982). This is just a reminder to get the whole story and to get it straight. Most questions on the list address the conceptual level: the concepts your patient has about the cause, treatment, or outcome of the illness, and the premises and logic the patient uses to work with those concepts. The last two questions deal with the affective level or personal meaning. Table 14 also presents some general categories of affective orien-

TABLE 13. Questions Defining the Conceptual Sphere:
Personal Meaning of Illness

Descriptive

1. How would you describe the problem that concerns you most?
2. What are the main difficulties this problem (sickness, illness, disease, misfortune) has caused for you?

Intellectual

3. What do you think is wrong, out of balance, or causing your problem?
4. What does the illness do to you? How does it work?
5. Why did it start when it did?
6. What kind of treatment do you think you should receive?
7. What are the results you hope for with treatment? Without treatment?
8. Apart from me (a medical doctor), who else can help you get better? What else can you do?

Affective

9. Why did you, as opposed to somebody else, get sick? And why now?
10. What do you fear most about your sickness?

---

tation toward illness, although often people's feelings about their sickness draw from more than one of these categories.

Beliefs about illness are frequently fragmented and not tightly integrated into a coherent system. People are constantly exposed to health information, on television and radio and in magazines and newspapers, from which a person may garner a variety of "facts" and opinions, some of which may be inconsistent with others. A person may learn that vitamin C cures the common cold, that vitamin E relieves impotence, or that chelation therapy removes calcium deposits from the lining of arteries. Some will consider these to be unrelated bits of information, while others will see them as part of a larger value system, such as the theory that most illness is caused by nutritional imbalance and is best treated by "natural" methods.

Here is an example of an elderly woman, blind from glaucoma, who had undergone chelation therapy and was explaining it to her new physician. Chelation involves the intravenous administration of EDTA, an agent that binds calcium and other cations, thus removing them from the

TABLE 14. Affective Meanings of Illness and Possible Patient Responses*

1. Illness as challenge
     Adapt actively
     Generates rational, task-oriented behavior
2. Illness as punishment
     Anxious, depressed, or angry
     May see opportunity for atonement
3. Illness as enemy
     Ready to fight, flee, or surrender
     Blame others
     Hostility, aggressiveness
4. Illness as weakness
     Shame, loss of control
     Conceal or deny illness
5. Illness as relief
     Reduces other obligations
6. Illness as strategy
     Strategic ploy to manipulate
     Dependent role, clinging
7. Illness as loss or damage
     Depression, hostility, resistance
     Prone to suicide
8. Illness as value
     Opportunity to reflect
     Expand personality
     Creative catalyst

*Adapted from Lipowski (1970).

body when it is excreted. It can be used to treat lead poisoning, for example. However, there is no sound evidence that it removes calcium from atherosclerotic plaques, and repeated intravenous treatments may be dangerous, as well as unnecessary and expensive. It is considered an unacceptable medical therapy. The physician has made this patient comfortable enough to describe why she did it, her feelings about it, and her evaluation of the outcome.

Dr: You had this creeping numbness and they didn't seem to know what to do about it?

Pt: Well, no, and then after the stroke, my back actually . . . I told you about the doctor, he said that it had already happened.

Dr: That your back had already, as you said, collapsed?

Pt: Well I didn't understand, I thought that my backbones would fall down. But what really happened was, I think, that the muscles that hold the bones together became like stretched out gumbands and for instance, like take an example, a car, you drive on an icy road. You want it to go one way and it goes another. I tried to go here but I had no control over my back. No control. I was talking to Dr. Smith but he would not do a thing, didn't do a thing. I mean it didn't seem to bother him at all. And then my bitter fear for my legs. Then, it came to the point, actually where my legs were just like a couple of logs. I would try to sleep at night and turn over and I would drag my legs.

Dr: Is that what made you afraid?

Pt: I was afraid, well I explained to Dr. Smith, "Look, Dr. Smith, there are people that lose the use of their legs and they go and use a wheelchair, but you got to have eyes to guide the wheelchair and I don't have that, what am I going to do?" But, like talking to the wall. Once he got very angry. "Do you think that if there would be something that would help you I wouldn't do it for you?" Well, as if it was a sin to even be concerned about myself. So anyway, well the situation was really awful, I was really fretting my mind all the time. I just lost the use of my eyes, next I lost the use of my legs, then what to do? All right? . . . After the chelation, these things never repeated. So, then I came to Dr. Brown and he said "I'll chelate you and you'll have no more strokes." So that's when I made up my mind, I have to go to the chelation—and it's better.

Dr: How often do you go now?

Pt: Well in the beginning it's good to go twice a week, but I've never been twice a week. It's not easy sitting four hours in one place. It takes three and a half to four hours.

Dr: You were afraid to tell me about this too, weren't you?

Pt: Yes, because you're not supposed to tell nobody about it.

Dr: Who says you're not supposed to tell?

Pt: The doctors. Well you should have seen Dr. Smith. He got mad. I felt so sick that time, he got so mad actually I don't know what was the matter with him. Like he was ready to get a nervous breakdown or something. *(Pauses.)* The thing is, it's so cruel. It's so cruel. Maybe it does do some good and if it does then why deprive a patient, just because of politics, that's not right. Come to Dr. Brown's office and its always filled up with chelating people, you know. So, I had once heard this woman telling, not to me, to others about a friend she knew. Now his legs became so bad they turned all black and his doctor advised him to have them amputated. Well that's a horrible prospect. But he, somebody told him about chelation, so he went and did it, and slowly the color came back in his legs and he started to be okay and he went back to work. This is hard to believe. So then he went to his doctor to show him and told him about the chelation but the doctor's response was, "if it was up to me I would still amputate." It's hard to believe such extreme cruelty.

Notice how the physician has found out about the chelation, despite the patient's proviso that "you're not supposed to tell." This doctor was faced with a patient who had spent much time and money on a form of treatment orthodox medicine considers completely worthless. Earlier physicians had let her down both by saying there was nothing to be done despite her "bitter fear for my legs," and by becoming angry if she told them about chelation. The main point for this doctor is to realize the patient feels better, her symptoms are largely resolved, and no academic discussion of quackery will alter that fact. The questions the physician will have to ask, himself or herself during the subsequent negotiation have nothing to do with the efficacy of chelation. The important questions are these: Are the beliefs really dangerous? Do they prohibit medical care that is actually necessary? Can I work within the patient's belief system to provide good medical care? Having answered these, the doctor must take the next step and arrive at a mutually acceptable course of action through the process of negotiation.

NEGOTIATION

Although patients cannot follow your advice unless they understand and remember it, noncompliance may also occur if they do not agree with it. So it is necessary to learn what the patient believes about what needs to be done for the illness. You can use this information to help the patient get well by attempting to change the patient's beliefs; by altering your therapeutic plan to accommodate them; or by reaching some intermediate, negotiated, therapeutic alliance. Negotiation is a process in which people use discussion and compromise to arrive at a settlement of some issue. In practice, negotiation is a way of optimizing patient compliance and is a sign of respect for the patient's autonomy. Once you have spoken with the patient and performed a physical examination, you will have some hypotheses, although you may remain uncertain about why the patient is ill or what the natural course of the patient's illness will be. You want to influence the patient's behavior, decrease his or her anxiety, and give the patient a better sense of control over the problem. How do you do this in the clinical interview?

Let us look at what several different authors consider crucial components of negotiation in medical practice. Benarde and Mayerson (1978) list the following components: (1) putting the patient at ease; (2) respect for the patient; (3) a positive attitude of the physician; (4) communication, which requires that you explain the information in understandable terms and provide feedback; (5) dealing adequately with the patient's response, particularly in terms of feelings; and (6) reaching a compromise position when there is conflict by a good faith "give-and-take." Brody (1980) wrote about the mutual participation model of doctor-patient interaction and lists these components: (1) a conducive atmosphere; (2) a method of ascertaining goals and expectations of the patient; (3) education of the patient about the problem and the treatment; and (4) eliciting from the patient informed suggestions, preferences, and disagreements. Heaton (1981) suggested that the spectrum of negotiation includes four subject areas: (1) agreement on what the clinical information really is; (2) consent for procedures or treatments; (3) agreement on the nature of the problem; and (4) agreement about what can or should be done.

Eraker and Politser (1982) outlined patient characteristics, physician traits and qualities of the doctor-patient relationship that facilitate or hinder compliance. They proposed a new way to understand and improve patient compliance that combines decision analysis, behavioral decision theory, and health beliefs. They stressed the importance of understanding the patient's "comprehension, decision-making processes and environment," and "acceptance of the diagnosis is particularly important because of the frequent occurrence of erroneous powerful health beliefs." These authors described certain physician tasks that influence the patient's behavior: (1) eliciting and respecting patients' concerns, and both patient and physician communicating their preferences; (2) evaluating the patient's comprehension and educating him or her in order to prevent that part of noncompliance that may be "nonvoluntary"; (3) learning about specific health beliefs, particularly those regarding perceived susceptibility and perceived severity; and (4) understanding the patient's perception of trade-offs between benefits and risks, and between quality and quantity of life.

All these authors have restated in different terms the familiar themes of respect, communication, beliefs, and expectations. You influence patients more when you respect them, when you communicate well with them, when you understand "where they're coming from," and so forth. An additional theme is that of uncertainty. The question of uncertainty is particularly important to emphasize for students just learning how to interview patients and negotiate with them. We presented elements of clinical judgment in the medical interview and discussed the problem of uncertainty in Chapter 7. The uncertainty that you experience is only partially because you are a beginner; much uncertainty is intrinsic to the doctor-patient interaction. From this perspective, you are negotiating not only to make the patient more likely to follow your suggestions or to understand your formulation, but also to achieve a better healing effect than could be obtained from a unilateral decision on your part combined with 100 percent patient compliance. This means that negotiation requires sharing your uncertainty with the patient. Gutheil and co-workers (1984) addressed this issue in the context of malpractice suit prevention. They speak of informed consent as

> . . . an interaction between physician and patient, a dialogue intended not only to satisfy a legal requirement but to do more as well. The real clinical opportunity offered by informed consent is that of transforming uncertainty from a threat to the doctor-patient alliance into the very basis upon which an alliance can be formed. . . . Note that our approach stresses the selection of what to say to patients rather than such advice as taking more time with patients or telling them more. In practice, less time is taken and more is understood: sound efficiency of communication, not mere volume of words, is the desideratum.

We will end this chapter with the following case example that demonstrates the interactive nature of clinical problem solving and the negotiation that occurs as new data are added. The case illustrates negotiation in both the "give-and-take" bargaining and the "maneuver to find a path" senses of the word. The elements of negotiation include presentation of evidence, the verification of evidence, its interpretation, the weighing of risks and benefits (including how physician and patient value different outcomes), and finally, the formulation of an agreement and plan of action.

A 25-year-old woman came into her doctor's office with the complaint of a severe and persistent vaginal itch. She expressed her distress, as well as summarizing her problem in her opening statement, which we encountered previously in Chapter 3:

> Pt: Well, I have a terrible vaginal itch, and I don't know whether it's from vaginitis or whether it's the urinary tract infection—

you know—ah, my regular doctor treated me for vaginitis
first . . .

Dr: That was Dr. X?

Pt: Ah, huh, then I, um, got a urinary tract infection, then the vaginitis came back, but during the whole ordeal I've never got no
relief.

We learn several important things about this patient from her opening
statement: she is suffering ("terrible," "ordeal," "no relief"), she is medically sophisticated ("vaginitis," "urinary tract infection"), and she is not
well educated in the sense of formal schooling ("I've never got no . . .").

The physician performs an examination, then leaves the room to examine a specimen under the microscope, returning with the news that the
infection is clearly caused by Trichomonas vaginalis and can be easily and
effectively treated with a single dose of eight pills. At this point, both
patient and physician agree on the nature of the problem: it is a Trichomonas infection. To the patient, the end of her suffering is in sight. The
physician begins to write out a prescription. But, seeing the name of the
drug as the physician writes it, the patient unexpectedly says:

Pt: Flagyl. You don't have any . . . there's nothing else you can take
besides Flagyl, huh?

Up until this point, it would appear as though the physician has made
not only an accurate diagnosis but also a correct decision about therapy
with which the patient will be happy. But the patient, instead of being
appropriately grateful for the physician's expertise, is not satisfied. The
negotiation begins:

Dr: It's the **best** for it.

Pt: Okay, but I might . . . well, I'll try it.

You could imagine a scenario here in which the physician simply says
"fine," and the patient is left to her own doubts about the drug, perhaps
taking it, perhaps not. But the physician, listening to her hesitation, replies:

Dr: What's the problem?

Pt: But I think I was allergic to that.

Dr: Why do you think that?

Pt: Because I remember taking Flagyl before, and it did something
. . . I think I broke out in hives or something.

Dr: Really?

Pt: But I'll try it, if I break out I'll let you know, but I think I did.

Dr: That's a worry . . . let me look at the record . . . it says here
that you were sensitive to ampicillin and sulfa . . . now could it
have been . . . Oh, it does say Flagyl . . .

> Pt: I think it was just hives. Maybe I've outgrown it.
>
> Dr: I don't want you to take it if you had hives from it.
>
> Pt: Well, maybe I'll have . . . I'll have outgrown it 'cause I think it's been a while back.
>
> Dr: *(Still looking through the chart)* Yeah, it does say Flagyl.

The patient actually begins with an interpretation ("allergic") of some past event associated with the drug. Physician and patient than exchange information, together trying to verify or refute that interpretation. The patient provides supporting evidence with the descriptive terms "hives," while the physician searches for other evidence by going through the patient's chart (she is new to this physician but had previously been seen in the same clinic). However, this is more than a simple discussion of evidence as we can see both patient ("I'll try it") and physician ("I don't want you to take it . . .") apparently on the verge of decisions, albeit opposite ones. Perhaps, seeing the physician's concern despite her willingness to risk hives, the patient offers a new interpretation to the data ("maybe I'll have outgrown it"). The physician then offers:

> Dr: What we **could** do is we could treat your husband and we could treat you with something else but . . .
>
> Pt: Well, if that's the best I want that . . .
>
> Dr: . . . most of the "something elses" aren't as effective.
>
> Pt: Well, I'll take Flagyl. It can only break me out in hives a day like . . . it'll probably go away in the morning.
>
> Dr: I would be kind of worried about that before prescribing it for you because you **could** get an even more serious reaction to it.

Data have been exchanged ("I was allergic"), verified ("hives," written record), and now reinterpreted ("I've outgrown it"). The patient, echoing the physician's "it's the **best**," rejects the notion of "something else" by reversing the implication of concession in her earlier statement on taking Flagyl ("well, I might try it"). In the context of the physician's earlier statement, "something else" would have to be seen as decidedly inferior. We are tiptoeing on a threshold-of-risk boundary: take Flagyl and get rid of the itch but risk an allergic reaction versus take something else and avoid the reaction but risk not curing the itch. Much of what the patient says in subsequent statements suggests that she places a higher value on getting rid of the itch than on avoiding an allergic reaction. The patient acknowledges that there is a risk involved but discounts it ("just hives"); the physician, on the other hand, stresses that the risk is more than that characterized by the patient ("you **could** get an even more serious reaction").

The decision has become problematic, and we begin to see both patient and physician engage in a dialogue regarding risks and benefits. Lacking the data to successfully value or weigh the risks, the physician returns to a discussion of the evidence, by turning again to the written record to find the supporting data for the diagnosis of allergy, while the patient in turn supplies additional details pointedly aimed at discrediting her own report of an allergic reaction:

Dr: . . . Uh, let me see what Dr. X said about that . . .

Pt: . . . I don't even think that Dr. X was here when I had that . . .

Dr: Dr. Y? Dr. Z? . . . because that may be why you've been treated with all this other stuff . . .

Pt: But they, I remember I told them it did that to me, it might notta been that.

Dr: But it does say you're allergic to it.

Pt: That's 'cause I **told** him that.

Dr: I've never heard anybody being allergic to it but it's . . .

Pt: That's what I'm saying it's . . .

Dr: . . . certainly possible . . .

Pt: . . . Probably what happened I broke out in hives in reaction to **other** things.

It is remarkable that the patient understands that the source of the data in question—or rather the interpretation in question—is herself (" 'cause I **told** him that") and that she may not be the most reliable interpreter of the evidence. Perhaps, if she is the source of the original interpretation, she can also be the source of a new interpretation. In the end, the physician is persuaded—to some extent. Note the ensuing discussion in which various outcomes are valued and a decision is reached:

Dr: Well, I'll tell you what I want you to do. Since you have taken a lot of drugs because of all these urinary infections . . .

Pt: . . . That might be why it's never left . . .

Dr: Uh hum . . .

Pt: . . . so I'd rather take the Flagyl . . .

Dr: . . . Well I'll tell you what I want you to do . . .

Pt: . . . It won't be your fault . . .

Dr: Well, I'm still the one that prescribes it. Let me tell you what I'd like you to do. I'd like you to take one pill out of your eight as a test dose. Okay? And if you have no reaction to it then we will hope it is safe to take the rest, though we can't know for sure.

Pt: Um hmm.

Dr: Today, just one, see what happens and if you have no reaction to it at all, then tomorrow take the remaining seven and have your husband take his eight. Okay?

Pt: Okay.

Dr: Okay? So if you are allergic we'll know . . .

Pt: Yeah, I'll get hives (ha ha).

Dr: Well, let's just be on the safe side, let's use a test dose . . . Okay? Because Trichomonas, while it's uncomfortable, it can't kill you so you know . . .

Pt: . . . It can drive you mad . . .

Dr: . . . I know, but the point is that we don't want to do anything that would be harmful to your health.

Although there was a lot of back-and-forth maneuvering, the physician takes ultimate responsibility for the decision ("I'm still the one that prescribes it"), but the decision is clearly influenced by the value the patient places on getting rid of the itch ("It can drive you mad"). The patient took the medication, had no reaction, and got rid of the itch. It is not difficult to imagine a different situation with a patient who had, perhaps, suffered more from hives, in which the negotiation would have resulted in a different outcome such as the prescribing of a somewhat less effective therapy.

We have addressed in this chapter the question of how you influence the patient's behavior through how you conduct the clinical interview. We have divided this influencing skill into three components for the sake of discussion, even though in practice they often flow together. **First,** the patient's understanding and recall of information must serve as a basis for any influence we might have. The patient cannot be compliant unless he or she knows what to do and how to do it. Moreover, the patient is not likely to be motivated to be compliant unless he or she knows why a particular plan is necessary and how it works. **Second,** the patient's own beliefs, conceptual framework, and affective orientation must all be considered in designing optimal therapy for your patient. Knowledge of this meaning sphere is essential for you to understand certain serious or chronic illnesses, as well as to promote optimal therapy for most significant illnesses. **Finally,** we discussed the role of negotiation in achieving an effective therapeutic outcome. Respect for the patient and knowledge of his or her beliefs would not necessarily help you to influence the patient unless you can use these while engaging in a process of negotiation to arrive at a plan of action.

CHAPTER 11

Symbolic Influence: The Placebo Effect

. . . It will be seen that minds do not *create* truth or falsehood. They create beliefs . . .

Bertrand Russell, *The Problems of Philosophy*

There is potentially a placebo effect of every interaction with every patient, and with every treatment we prescribe. Knowledge of placebo effects has grown rapidly during the last generation; we are now aware that they occur almost everywhere we look in medicine, and we must therefore design our experiments ever more elegantly to avoid them. The practicing physician is left in a quandary. If placebo effects are always operative in medicine, why not simply ignore them and focus on specific treatment that we can "add" to this underlying phenomenon? Isn't there something unethical and misleading about too much reliance or concentration on the placebo effect? Even if a physician acknowledges the placebo effect in his or her practice and begins to study it, what can he or she do to change it? These questions leave the doctor with a general feeling that the placebo effect may be real and it may be universal, but it is a mild and transient phenomenon, perhaps important but not controllable in medical practice.

This attitude toward the placebo effect is at least partly a matter of semantics. For "placebo effect" to be more thoroughly appreciated and used by practicing physicians (as opposed to being studied by researchers), we must first remove the idea that we are dealing with a subset of medications or procedures, or with a kind of deception, and then acknowledge that we are speaking about a whole array of greater or lesser, harmful or beneficial influences rather than a single effect. We object to the conceptual and emotional baggage of placebo effect. That is why we prefer the term "symbolic healing" and use it in the context of a general model in which any medical treatment has a symbolic influence, as well as focal and behavioral influences (see Chapter 12).

In earlier chapters, we commented on the fact that patients will frequently tell you that their pain or other symptoms got better just before coming in to see the doctor. Others will come back after a diagnostic x-ray, before you have prescribed any treatment, and explain how much better they are feeling. These and other phenomena will be part of your experience with the ordinary medical interview, and as you begin to take responsibility for patient care, you will see many other instances in which your interaction with the patient seems to promote healing. You will also, undoubtedly, experience times in which your interactions lead to increased patient anxiety and a worsening of symptoms. Both of these effects will occur with patients who have "physical" illness and disease; we are not focusing here on patients who have neurotic symptoms or somatization disorders. This chapter introduces you to the concept that you can enhance symbolic healing while you are taking a medical history or doing an ordinary interview and so become actively involved in a process that Shapiro termed "iatroplacebogenesis" (Shapiro, 1971).

PLACEBOS AND PLACEBO EFFECTS

Physicians usually consider placebo effects only in one of three restrictive senses: (1) the actual treatment of a patient with a "placebo" or "sugar pill" under certain circumstances; (2) a nonspecific influence that must be controlled as a prerequisite for performing adequate clinical trials of new therapy; or (3) a rather vague explanation for unanticipated therapeutic effects. Each of these notions captures some element of truth about placebo effects but only in a limited manner. It will be helpful to consider these ideas in a little more detail, before turning to the skills of "iatroplacebogenesis," or symbolic healing.

Sugar Pills

One frequent attitude you will encounter in the hospital is the concept that placebo relief of pain or another symptom somehow suggests that the symptom is not "real." This is the "sugar pill" sense of the term. Physicians and nurses have a striking lack of knowledge about placebo potency. For example, in one study most doctors felt that a placebo relief indicates that chest pain is noncardiac in origin (Goodwin, Goodwin, and Vogel, 1979). Surveys suggest that hospital personnel frequently still use placebo as a tool to differentiate functional from organic pain (Grey and Flynn, 1981; Goodwin, Goodwin, and Vogel, 1979). But what do the data really tell us about this phenomenon?

Beginning with the landmark work of Beecher (1955) and Lasagna and co-workers (1954), studies of placebo treatments have most often concerned modification of symptoms, such as postoperative pain, peptic ulcer pain, arthritic pain, headache, angina pectoris, sea sickness, anxiety, and depression. These are all clear-cut medical problems. Other observers have documented the physiologic actions of placebos using objective measurements: lowering of blood pressure, preventing postoperative complications, healing of peptic ulcers, decreasing gastric acid production, preventing asthmatic attacks, lowering blood sugar, and decreasing inflammation. In any given treatment situation, about 35 percent of patients will respond with a positive placebo effect. This is remarkably constant among studies and is not "imaginary."

Much conflicting data regarding characteristics of the placebo effect arise from studies that focus on only one aspect of the situation rather than on the treatment context as a whole; for example, studies of pills given under supposedly standardized situations or studies of patients' personalities. We have conflicting data, for example, on the time course or natural history of placebo effects. Beecher and Lasagna found that 53 percent of patients with severe postoperative pain responded to one dose of placebo, 40 percent consistently to two or three doses, and only 15 percent consistently to four or more doses. This suggests a wearing-off phenomenon. On the other hand, studies of ulcer healing or the duration of symptoms in chronic disease suggest a more sustained effect. Sarles and co-workers (1977) charted mean duration of symptoms in the placebo groups of various duodenal ulcer studies. They found that placebo was substantially more effective than "no treatment" in reducing the total duration of peptic ulcer symptoms.

In the 1950s investigators assumed that people of a certain personality configuration, those with high "suggestibility," would consistently respond to placebos but that people with other personality types would not. Subsequently, extensive studies have failed to identify such a "placebo responder" personality. Generally, age, sex, intelligence quotient, and alcohol consumption have not been associated with placebo response. Certain other characteristics, considered individually, do have some predictive value. Various observers have characterized patients whose symptoms were relieved by placebos as more likely than nonresponders to (1) demonstrate enthusiastic, verbal, extroverted behavior patterns; (2) have completed higher education; (3) be nonsmokers; (4) work in a "better" occupation; and (5) hold "medium," as opposed to very high or very low expectations about getting well. Moertl and associates (1976) postulated a model consistent with most of these data. It suggests that people more likely to respond to placebos regularly are those with a high level of personal responsibility, and those in positions that demand independent performance. In other words, those who have a sense of internal control and who approach the illness situation realistically are most likely to obtain relief from placebo therapy. This certainly calls into question the use of placebos as a test for "crocks."

Moreover, prescribing a placebo treatment almost always involves misleading the patient, at least by implication, into thinking he or she is receiving a specific drug treatment. This practice, paradoxically, is most often used in cases when it is least likely to be effective. In cases of chronic pain, for example, when the physician has reason to believe that the pain is psychogenic rather than originating from a physical lesion, the physician might prescribe a saline injection rather than an analgesic. This frequently happens with patients perceived to be hostile or demanding in the hospital setting. The empirical data, however, suggest that severe pain is more likely to respond to a placebo than mild pain, and that physical pain is more likely to respond than psychogenic pain. Consequently, a positive placebo response in the setting described might actually be counterintuitive: it might suggest "real" organic origin as opposed to an emotional origin for the pain.

This conscious use of inert placebo involves deception and cannot be justified in medical practice. More commonly, rather than using an inert placebo pill, physicians give active drugs while still having a placebo intent. For example, a patient may complain of leg pain, which the doctor ascertains to be caused by poor arterial circulation. While the physician may realize there are no effective drugs to improve circulation in such cases, he or she may prescribe a drug that was once thought to be "good for circulation" but is now known to be ineffective. The doctor prescribes it simply because the patient expects some treatment. In such a case, the medication must really be considered a placebo, even though it may have specific effects in other situations. The intent is to deceive the patient, and the practice is unethical.

This class of cases is not too far removed from another class in which symptomatic treatment is given but the patient may believe he or she has received specific treatment. A person may be quite ill with a self-limited disease, such as acute viral gastroenteritis, and the physician merely prescribes treatment to ameliorate symptoms until the infection resolves on its own. Since ill people often do not make the distinction between a set of symptoms and the "entity" that underlies those symptoms, the difference between symptomatic and definitive therapy may be at least partially obscure, **even if the physician** pays reasonable attention to describing the actual effect of the medicine.

This latter situation, the (inadvertent) use of symptomatic drugs as "placebos," brings us closer to understanding how pervasive placebo effects are. The nature of the patient's expectations and the manner in which physicians meet or do not meet those expectations may influence therapy. Patient expectations may be based on mistaken beliefs about illness and about what should be done for illness. It may well be unrealistic and undesirable for the physician to alter those beliefs substantially in many illness situations. On the other hand, it is unethical for a physician to contribute to those mistaken beliefs, such as by prescribing medication that he or she knows to be without specific efficacy.

Clinical Trials

The second commonly appreciated role of placebo is in clinical trials to evaluate the efficacy of new therapy. In such studies, after the investigator obtains informed consent, one group of patients, usually selected randomly, receives the potentially active drug, while another group receives an inert substance that looks and tastes the same and is given according to the same schedule. This procedure controls for the placebo effect so that the net, specific action of the drug is only the difference in positive outcome between those receiving the drug and those receiving placebo. If an analgesic controls pain in 75 percent of the patients and placebo controls it in 40 percent, we might conclude, assuming our test was powerful enough, that the analgesic is significantly more effective than placebo, or even state that it was almost twice as effective as placebo. However, we could not conclude that the analgesic is specifically responsible for relieving the pain in 75 percent of the patients. Thus, by considering the placebo effect in the **design** of modern clinical trials, we try to eliminate it as a factor for explaining our positive results.

Our belief in placebo as an element of good experimental methodology fixes squarely on the requirement that "groups be identical in every way, except for our independent variable—the experimental treatment." The additional requirement that both patients and physicians be "blinded" to the actual treatment given tidies up the design still further. This focus on **sameness** as a goal in itself to facilitate analysis fails to look beyond the method to explore **why** sameness and placebo controls are so important. Interestingly, this emphasis on placebo as simply a factor in experimental design can lead to the ethically questionable practice of employing placebos in a trial when an alternate, accepted form of treatment is available for the disease. Under those circumstances, the researcher should compare any experimental medication with the current standard of therapy, whatever it may be. If the standard is already moderately effective, perhaps curing 70 percent of patients, it will be very difficult to demonstrate a significant advantage of a new drug, because it would require an enormous number of subjects to produce enough power to demonstrate a statistically significant difference, even if the new drug cured 90 percent of the patients. Thus, researchers might prefer to offer placebo, knowing that then they are more likely to end up with a "positive" trial than if they offer standard treatment.

Even in the rigid format of clinical trials, however, the placebo effect is not a constant: it varies with the subject's expectations. Those patients who first receive an active drug such as aspirin in a crossover trial protocol are more likely to respond to placebo later when their treatment is switched during the second part of the protocol. Thus, placebo response can be upgraded by prior experience with an active agent (Moertl, 1976). This suggests a conditioning effect. A simple set of instructions given to subjects may also serve as a "placebo" that facilitates the appearance of a specific drug effect. For example, in a trial of phenmetrazine versus placebo for appetite suppression, neither treatment led to significantly reduced appetite in uninstructed, blinded subjects. However, when subjects in both groups were told that appetite suppression might occur after taking the pills, those receiving phenmetrazine subsequently ingested about 220 calories less during their evening meals, as compared with those taking placebo (Penick and Hinkle, 1964).

Other studies suggest that drugs that have some noticeable symptomatic effect may be more potent "placebos" than inert substances. Thompson (1982) reviewed 75 clinical trials of tricyclic antidepressant therapy for depression. He found that in 43 of 68 trials using inert placebos, the tricyclic drug was superior in ameliorating depressive symptoms; but in 6 of 7 trials using atropine as an "active" placebo, there was no difference between the treatments in clinical outcome. Atropine itself is known not to be a specific antidepressant drug. It does, however, produce clear side effects, so that the patient knows he or she is taking a "potent" medication. The physiologic effects of atropine raise expectations that the drug is active, and therefore make its placebo effect more powerful. This is analogous to the situation we often encounter (discussed earlier), in which symptomatic treatment, although intended only for symptom suppression, actually results in quicker healing and more patient satisfaction.

Unorthodox Healing

The third connotation of the placebo effect is that of explaining unorthodox or unexpected treatment effects. We may apply it to chiropractic or megavitamin therapy, to faith healing or Christian Science, to indigenous medicine of other cultures or to ancient medicine in our own. This is a case of recognizing the mote in your brother's eye, while failing to see the beam in your own. If such healing effects, in fact, occur in unorthodox healing, the same factors must also occur within the orthodox biomedical system. Although we recognize the placebo effect as a phenomenon, we tend always to ascribe ordinary results in ordinary medical care to the specific or "focal" effects of our interventions.

Our formulary of medical treatments would be quite small were we to restrict it to those medications proven effective by randomized controlled trials, and for which the mechanisms of action are entirely understood. We know, however, that the biomedical model is a robust one, supported in a variety of ways (for example, in vitro experiments, animal models, clinical trials, and epidemiologic surveys) by a number of different disciplines (for example, molecular biology, histochemistry, pharmacokinetics, and gross anatomy). Concepts "fit" together and form a matrix of understanding. Thus, when we make an unexpected observation, such as a presumed drug effect in illness, we can suggest a number of different hypotheses to explain the effect, all within the range of admissible hypotheses that "fit" our understanding of how the body works. Alternate healing systems, such as chiropractic, homeopathy, or religious healing, present treatments and explanations that fall outside this range. The placebo effect or the power of "expectant faith," as described by Jerome Frank (1975), is the only point of contact commonly acknowledged by medical practitioners.

Our model of the healing act provides another way to analyze patient response to such unorthodox systems. The overt treatment provided by chiropractors, for example, is likely to have some **focal** benefit for patients with musculoskeletal problems, particularly those of the neck and back. While chiropractic's theory of vertebral subluxation and nerve root interference is at odds with biomedical knowledge, the relief of symptoms by spinal adjustment is supported by clinical experience and by some controlled investigations (Coulehan, 1985). Chiropractors can also induce some **behavioral** change by encouraging exercise programs and dietary modification. Their art can produce a strong symbolic healing vector through such features as validating the patient's suffering, understandable explanation of the cause of the illness, enthusiastic faith in the outcome of treatment, and sustained physical contact or "laying-on-of-hands." These effects can be synergistic, as when the relief of back pain by spinal adjustment tends to confirm to the patient the chiropractor's explanations and suggestions. This may well lead to some symbolic healing effect for manipulative treatment when it is subsequently applied to a type of problem, such as dyspepsia, on which it is unlikely to have any focal effect.

Another example of such potentiation is the use of ascorbic acid for the prevention and treatment of colds. Various clinical trials have suggested small positive responses to supplements ranging from 250 mg to several grams daily. Yet, in the aggregate, the studies demonstrate no consistent, clinically significant reduction in morbidity (Coulehan, 1979). However, ascorbic acid does appear to have some antihistaminic activity in high doses and, thus, might cause sensitive persons to experience enough change in their bodily sensations that it could serve as an "active" placebo (see earlier). In this case, a clinically insignificant **focal** vector might supplement the **symbolic** vector associated with vitamins and "natural" treatment in many people's minds.

Christian Science presents an example in which there is no evident **focal** vector of therapy at all. From a medical perspective, it is entirely a system of mind control, in which the ill person systematically learns that sickness, and even the body itself, is unreal (Talbot, 1983). We are spiritual beings, and the physical reality we see is merely an illusion or dream. Consequently, the sick person is simply in error, and becoming well is equivalent to "unlearning" that error. Such a radical belief has a strong personal impact on those able to accept it and also stimulates a **behavioral** change in that the person adopts a systematic program of "prayer" to achieve his goal.

Some healing acts in medicine, such as the therapeutic effect of "getting tests done" or, for that matter, of a "routine" history and physical also appear to have no focal component. On the other hand, acts that are focally appropriate may lead to dissatisfaction, disability, and increased suffering. There must, of course, be a common denominator—a final common pathway—among the vectors of healing. If we are willing to accept the efficacy of Christian Science in at least some of the many thousands of illnesses its practitioners treat, we must postulate that the personal or symbolic vector contributes to healing through some intermediate, physiologic steps. The symbolic factor must become instrumental in the same way that a focal treatment is instrumental, by influencing biochemical systems. But how does this occur?

The healing encounter is effective when it reduces the suffering of illness, whether this be through treating disease, treating symptoms, or helping to transform the illness's symbolic meaning, thus allowing the patient to have less anxiety and more control. The generic situation is one in which expectation of healing triggers a physiologic response, leading to alteration in symptoms or even to alteration in the homeostatic state that sustains the illness. Expectation is a function of interpretation in the light of prior beliefs; in other words, it results from the **meaning** of a situation and somehow alters biochemical systems. This may possibly occur through generation or release of neurohormones and other, as yet unidentified substances. It is not unreasonable to assume that placebo-type influences, although they always have some effect, may under certain circumstances have major effects in altering the homeostatic system.

Doctor-Patient Interaction

These three meanings for "placebo effect"—sugar pills, control in clinical trials, and unorthodox healing—converge to a universal phenomenon that occurs to some extent, to help or to heal, in every doctor-patient interaction. The doctor, in an ordinary interview, even while taking the patient's history, can begin to help the patient feel better.

One review article presented evidence from 34 different studies that had shown important beneficial effects of "psychological interventions" for patients after acute myocardial infarction or prior to surgery (Mumford, Schlesinger, and Glass, 1982). The intervention described in each study was a standardized one for patients in a given group and did not take into account the individual's beliefs, coping style, or clinical circumstances. Nonetheless, "psychological interventions" such as patient education and emotional support led to better outcomes in the study groups. Similar interventions have been advanced as demonstrating the placebo effect in earlier literature (Egbert et al, 1964). It seems reasonable that further tailoring these interventions to the specific healing act would, in fact, be substantially more beneficial. Let us consider three interventions for a man who has had an acute myocardial infarction: careful explanation of the coronary care process so that he knows what to expect; brief emotional-support visits with little cognitive content, but conveying empathic understanding and respect; and a careful interview eliciting the patient's attributions, orientation, and expectations with regard to his illness. These could easily be additive or even synergistic. If each of these effects is explained by a placebo response, there must be multiple types of placebo responses. The same patient who had all of these interventions from a conscientious coronary care staff might also be given a nitroglycerin tablet when he complained of chest pain, which, unknown to the nurse, was actually due to pericarditis rather than to ischemia. If the pain improved as a result of nitroglycerin, the placebo effect could again be invoked, in this case with its more traditional connotation.

It is obvious that whatever is beneficial in these various interventions must come about through a variety of different mechanisms. Insofar as the interventions reduce sympathetic nervous activity, they are just as **focal** as beta-blockers in treating symptoms. Insofar as they engage the patient in his or her own care, they are **behavioral**. Insofar as they reduce the patient's anxiety and improve his or her understanding and perception of control, they are personal or **symbolic**. The psychologic interventions reviewed in Mumford and associates (1982)—empathic listening, general emotional support, clear communication—are other uses for the same skills that lead to objective and precise data collection.

We discussed in Chapter 10 three aspects of influencing behavioral change: accurate transmittal of information so that the patient understands it and can recall it; investigation of the patient's beliefs about what caused his or her illness and what might be done about it; and the process of negotiation. To do these well, the physician must have mastered the basic skills of respect, genuineness, and empathy (Chapter 2). He or she must also have developed facility with attending and responding, skills embodied in the structure of the interview itself (Chapters 3 through 6).

Here we are concentrating on another aspect of influencing patients, helping them by changing the personal meaning of their illness and thereby reducing their level of anxiety and increasing their sense of control over the illness. Here are two examples in which the doctor was using her skills to create a therapeutic symbolic influence:

CASE 1:

Dr: There's no serious threat to your health right now. This pain, I think, is related to the spasms that you have in the muscle there in the chest.

Pt: Yeah.

Dr: And in the back, and it's probably related to your arthritis, too.

Pt: I was wonderin'. I said to my friend, I said, I wonder when it was hurtin' like that, when it would grab, I said could that be arthritis, too? Because I know a friend that I worked with, we worked in dampness all those years, our hands were wet. And lots of times the floors were wet. And, um, with age it's just catchin' up with me.

Dr: But you know I think that the worry, too, contributes to the pain.

Pt: Mm mm.

Dr: Because any time the muscles and the joints aren't so well to begin with and you have worries, everything hurts worse and the muscles tend to be more tense. And you have a muscle right under the skin, here in your head, that may be causing your headaches. *(Demonstrates to patient.)* So I'd like to start you on the Motrin, but I'd also like to deal with some of these worries that you have. To see whether we can get you feeling **better**.

Pt: Mm hm.

Dr: . . . As far as the worries go.

Pt: Well, I just have to, I'm tryin' to, um, throw it off. I believe in goin' out and I pray and ask Him to help me to not worry, put it in His hands.
(Doctor nods.)

Pt: Because there's nothing I can do about it. And I, um, through life tend to worry about every little thing. Even I wasn't doing too well in school 'til I made up my mind what I can't do is worry.

Dr: *(Nods.)* Right.

Pt: Give up some of it, then I started bein' an A student, which I could have been **all** the time if I hadn't worried.

Dr: Well, you're certainly a person that's done a lot to help yourself.

CASE 2:

Pt: Lately, Lord, I keep getting this pain in my arm and short of breath and turn purple, you know, I get sorta scared, you know . . . Like a couple of times, you know I called the emergency room 'cause I was gettin' pains in my arm and my God the girl

Dr: that answered said "Get in here right away." "You get into this Emergency Room," you know.

Dr: Yes.

Pt: But I hated to just come right away, well, you can't just come right away. You gotta get stuff ready, you know, and I says I don't know what to do. She says "if it was me, I'd know what I'd do." You know, she says to get right in here. Well, in three minutes you can have a heart attack and be gone. And I get, you know, scared and I say should I go over or shouldn't I go over? And I just wait and try to sit it out and there's quite a few times that I just sit it out. You know.

Dr: Your heart is fine. I think what's been causing your symptoms is acid from your stomach sneaking back up into your esophagus. Here, I'll draw you a picture.

(And later . . .)

Pt: Yeah, so I took the two Mylanta. Thank God I did get better, 'cause I didn't wanna be callin' the paramedics. Jesus, I hate to do that unless I hafta. But I didn't know what the hell to do. What the hell's the matter with me? You know, gettin' short of breath like that, I don't like to get that way.

Dr: Well, I think now you have a better idea what to do.

Pt: Yeah, thank God that Mylanta relieves it a little bit. What's causin' the dizziness, you know?

Dr: It may be from that virus you had. I don't think it's anything that will stay with you. Now that you can control the chest pain some, maybe the dizziness will be easier for you to handle.

Each of these vignettes demonstrates how the doctor was attempting to influence the patient by enhancing the patient's sense of control. In one way, this was a behavioral influence dealing with specific activities (taking Mylanta, relaxing muscles). However, in another way, the influence was directed toward promoting healing by reinforcing the patient's positive self-image ("You're certainly a person that's done a lot to help yourself" and "Now that you can control the chest pain maybe the dizziness will be easier for you to handle.")

CHAPTER 12

The Healing Act

The faith that heals, heals not through argument but by contagion. But to heal, faith must have substance. A speculative balance of probability is not enough. The faith that heals must have deep roots in the personality of the healer.

W. R. Houston, *The Doctor Himself as a Therapeutic Agent*

What is the outcome of your interaction with a patient? What have you achieved when you walk out after completing the history and physical examination? Of course, you have established a large part of the medical data base for that patient; moreover, you have initiated a diagnostic strategy. In this book we have stressed the data collection and hypothesis testing aspects of your medical interview. Your goal, in that respect, is to achieve the right diagnosis and, ultimately, to prescribe the right treatment. You then communicate all this to the patient during the termination phase of the interview.

In practice, however, any medical interaction has a more complex outcome than diagnosis alone. When you walk out of the hospital room, or when the patient walks out of your office, you will have in some way **influenced** that patient. Of course, you intend to influence the patient's illness through arriving at the correct diagnosis and prescribing adequate treatment. But you influence patients in two other important ways as well. **First**, you influence their subsequent behavior by asking them to undertake diagnostic studies, follow a regimen of medication, return for subsequent office visits, stop smoking cigarettes, or embark on an exercise program. When patients change their behavior in these ways, we say they are "compliant" or that they follow our medical advice. Clearly, the best diagnosis and treatment in the world will be useless without some of this influence on behavior. We discussed this type of influence in Chapter 10.

186

Second, we influence how patients think and feel. We may cause some change in a patient's concept of what the illness is and what it means, and thereby reduce his or her anxiety or, alternatively, increase it. The patient may walk away relieved or sorely distressed. We may have somehow started to diminish his or her burden of suffering, or added to it iatrogenic suffering. It is this sort of influence that Michael Balint, the British psychiatrist, had in mind when he taught that "the doctor is the drug" (Balint, 1972) and what more recent observers refer to as the "placebo effect" of doctor-patient interactions (Brody, 1982). We discussed these influences in Chapter 11.

How do you maximize the chance that your influence on the patient will be positive or beneficial? In this book we have been concerned with the skills of medical interviewing, particularly history taking. Yet, what you do and the way you do it as you take the history will have multiple effects: good technique may maximize the objectivity and precision of the data on which you base your hypotheses, but at the same time good technique may result in the patient's following your advice and leaving your office with a sense of well-being and relief. It may not be possible to dissect and examine each different aspect of your influence in a given situation, but for teaching purposes we have considered separately the features of influence on patient compliance and on the placebo effect. You bring concepts and skills together in the process of negotiation. Now we will present a model and look in more detail at the doctor's influence on patients—an influence that actually begins with taking the history as the first step in what we call "the healing act."

A MODEL OF THE DOCTOR-PATIENT INTERACTION

After a patient has seen a doctor, that patient is likely to be changed in some way. While the person may or may not have received the specific help sought, **something** relevant to his or her health care is different. The influence may well be quite small, yet it is potentially observable. The patient may know more about his or her problem or may have received misinformation. The patient's anxiety may be decreased or increased, or replaced by a quality of anxiety different from that which brought him or her to the doctor. His or her symptoms may be decreased or increased, or replaced by new symptoms. The patient's opinion of doctors in general, or of one doctor in particular, may well be altered. Sick and suffering persons experience the world differently than well people (Cassell, 1976). They are frequently in a "crisis situation" when they seek medical help, a time when small interventions might have significant outcomes. Among all these outcomes, relevant ones cluster into beneficial (symptom reduction, anxiety reduction, satisfaction, compliance) or harmful (symptom increase, anxiety increase, dissatisfaction, lack of compliance) groups. In other words, any doctor-patient interaction is likely, at least in some small way, to influence the suffering of a sick person.

The net direction and magnitude of this influence is determined by the simultaneous contributions of three factors which we have illustrated in Figure 3. Each factor or category of influence is displayed as an axis in this representation of a three-dimensional figure. The most helpful or healing interactions are those with strongly positive focal, behavioral, and symbolic influences; in such cases the net vector places them in the upper left-hand section of the figure. The most harmful or negative interactions are those in which the sum of these three influences can be plotted in the lower right-hand section. The following two cases will help to illustrate what we mean in naming these axes focal, behavioral, and symbolic.

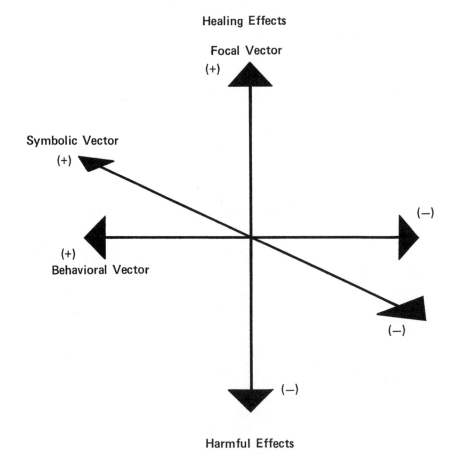

FIGURE 3. A model of the healing act: factors influencing the net vector of doctor-patient interaction.

Case 1. A young woman came to the Health Center because of mid-thoracic back pain radiating to her left anterior chest. At the first visit her doctor found a "trigger point" in the right paravertebral muscles at the T4 level, and he injected the area with a local anesthetic solution. She and the doctor also discussed her episodic attacks, which included tachycardia, weakness, dizziness, and breathlessness, along with exacerbation of chest pain. She had had an extensive medical work-up for these symptoms at another hospital, including an exercise electrocardiogram and an echocardiogram, both of which were normal. After the "trigger point" injection, she had muscle soreness in the area for several days, but no sharp chest or back pain during months of follow-up.

She subsequently said that her vigilant focusing on the pain had increased her anxiety and precipitated panicky reactions to it. Once she recognized that the symptom **could** be controlled, she no longer suffered, and eagerly sought to control her own symptoms through a graduated exercise program recommended by her doctor.

Case 2. A middle-aged man had chronic back and neck pain that left him disabled since his long bout of cryptococcal meningitis 10 years previously. He came in to the Health Center with a specific new pain in the epigastric region, which he had experienced for three months. His previous physician had concluded the new complaint was just another instance of the patient's chronic socialization around somatic language, and dismissed it. He prescribed analgesics. Although the symptom complex was atypical for peptic ulcer, the new doctor decided to order a thorough evaluation, which included an upper GI x-ray series. This proved to be normal. Nonetheless, the patient returned to the office on an up-beat note, saying his pain was better and that it was probably related to his chronic problems. He said he "understood" these, but when the new pain began he felt he might have something "serious like cancer." His brother had recently died of heart disease, and a niece had died of leukemia during the preceding Christmas holiday. The patient's further care included a regular program of relaxation techniques, supported by scheduled medical visits. The diagnostic x-rays, in this case, may have symbolized a level of concern on the part of his physician that helped relieve his suffering.

We call a specific expected alteration of pathophysiology, using treatment directed to the biochemical, cellular, or structural levels, the **focal vector** of healing. Theoretically, this aspect of medicine does not depend on dynamics of doctor-patient interaction but rather on pharmacology, biochemistry, surgery, and the characteristics of the patient's disease process.

In Case 1 the work of the focal vector was done by an injection of a local anesthetic into a small area of muscle spasm. The injection was "focal" insofar as it worked directly (focally) to influence biologic function. This vector, in other cases, might be the bacteriocidal effects of penicillin, the surgery that removes an infected gallbladder, or the lowered cardiac oxygen requirements induced by a beta-blocker medication. A treatment may serve as a focal vector even when the explanation for its effect is unknown, as in the "trigger point" example, or when the explanation given for its effectiveness is at odds with biomedical knowledge, as is possibly the case with spinal adjustment performed by chiropractors (Coulehan, 1985). Case 2 illustrates that satisfactory outcomes may occur in the apparent absence of any focal component. The patient felt better and was satisfied, although no specific treatment for his epigastric pain was given.

The second influence on outcome in Figure 3, the **behavioral vector**, refers to those elements of the doctor-patient interaction that modify the extent to which the patient adheres to therapy, follows advice, or undertakes any behavioral modification to resolve a problem. Compliance with treatment depends on patient satisfaction, coping style, health beliefs, the attribution of symptoms, and the amount of information recalled regarding what to do and how to do it. The doctor-patient interaction can be used to modify several of these factors in ways that might promote adherence to therapy or, on the other hand, make compliance less likely. The young woman in the first case pursued a successful exercise program as a result of a positive behavioral factor. The program itself, insofar as it strengthened her muscles and improved underlying muscle tone, was focal treatment; but the motivation to perform it was a behavioral factor. In Case 2 the patient's subsequent adherence to a schedule of regular clinic visits for supportive care constituted a behavioral healing effect.

The third component of a healing act is the **symbolic vector**, or personal interpretation of what goes on between doctor and patient. We use the term "symbolic" to designate what the illness means to the patient, how he or she integrates it into life experience and plans. This personal meaning may include a mixture of several "meanings": (1) some basic explanation of the symptom in terms of prior knowledge or experience ("folk physiology"); (2) possible medical labels, especially dreaded diseases like cancer; (3) preconscious or subconscious metaphoric understanding of the symptoms; (4) an assessment of illness consequences on life, ego integrity, functioning, and other family members; and (5) a fundamental attitude toward illness and suffering (a challenge, a random event, a punishment, and so on). The doctor's influence on personal meaning may reduce the underlying anxiety associated with sickness and lead the patient to experience a sense of control that decreases suffering. Donald Sandner, a Jungian psychiatrist, expressed an important facet of the need for symbolic healing when he wrote "The doctor . . . who works with people in distress . . . learns that man can accept a tremendous amount of legitimate suffering;

what he cannot accept is suffering that has no purpose. To be endured and accepted, suffering must be given a meaning" (Sandner, 1979). The symbolic vector adds individual, often idiosyncratic, elements to sociocultural meanings; and it recognizes multiple and sometimes conflicting "meanings" that any one person may hold for a given illness.

The symbolic vector follows from those activities of the doctor and interpretations by the patient that yield what Shapiro termed "iatroplacebogenesis" (Shapiro, 1971), although, as discussed in Chapter 11, we prefer to avoid its identification with the term "placebo." In both the young woman with chest pain and the man with epigastric pain, the doctor succeeded in altering the patient's understanding of what the illness meant, and in giving the patient some control over it. These were examples of a beneficial symbolic vector.

On first view, it appears that at least two components, the behavioral and symbolic, go hand in hand, with behavioral change being an outward manifestation of symbolic change or "iatroplacebogenesis." However, these two are not inextricably related. It is possible, for example, that a hypertensive patient may have an excellent relationship with his physician and believe that his medical care has resulted in improved health, yet hardly ever take his antihypertensive medication. He may have noticed that the pills resulted in sexual dysfunction and, consequently, stopped taking them while not considering this fact important enough to tell his physician. Alternatively, he may have a belief system that places more value on decreasing "tension" in his life than on the long-term use of drugs. In such a case, the symbolic factor may be effective, while the behavioral influence (for example, compliance) is minimal. A second patient with hypertension may, because of his obsessive style or his tendency to submit to any authority figure, take the same medication regularly despite the fact that he has a poor relationship with his doctor and is dissatisfied with the outcome of medical care. Ordinarily, however, symbolic and behavioral influences do overlap, so that an approach to interviewing and patient care that enhances the one will usually also enhance the other.

The focal, behavioral, and symbolic vectors are interdependent and result in a unitary healing act. Your treatment is the net outcome for the patient; it is not simply the focal prescription. Without effective attention to the woman's symptoms in Case 1, the doctor likely would not have been able to engage her in a back care program. We would argue that neither the injection nor the exercises would have been effective had he not assisted in changing her feeling of control over the illness.

INTERACTION AND IATROGENESIS

The net influence of a doctor-patient interaction is not always beneficial. Physicians intend to relieve the burden of their patient's suffering and find it painful themselves when they fail to do so. Yet we sometimes cause symptoms through the focal effects of our treatment. Physical iatrogenesis includes the side effects of drugs, symptoms of drug interactions, and the physical risks and pain associated with diagnostic and surgical procedures. This can occur, as we noted in Chapter 7, when ineffective or even harmful treatments achieve popularity, as did irradiation for enlarged thymus glands in the 1940s, diethylstilbesterol to prevent miscarriages in the 1950s, or gastric freezing for peptic ulcer in the early 1960s. Such organized iatrogenesis is still likely to be happening today as we engage in what William Roe (1984) terms "therapeutic fantasies."

Physicians can also create suffering through the behavioral and symbolic influences they have on patients. The following case illustrates a vicious circle of iatrogenic suffering, which sometimes occurs in medical care.

> **Case 3.** RD was a 64-year-old woman with atherosclerotic heart disease who had had coronary artery bypass surgery for angina when she was 58 years old. She began to experience episodes of left retroorbital headache associated with blepharospasm. She was referred to a neurologist who thought the episodes were inconsistent with transient ischemic attacks, yet ordered an evaluation of her carotid artery flow, which revealed high-grade obstruction in the left internal carotid artery. The noninvasive studies were confirmed by arteriogram. She came to the hospital for possible endarterectomy, but upon admission experienced severe substernal chest pain.
>
> RD transferred to the cardiology service where an acute myocardial infarct was ruled out, and she subsequently had exercise stress testing, MUGA scan, and coronary angiography. The latter showed two patent grafts with no progression in her underlying atherosclerotic lesions. The cardiologist said that RD's bout of chest pain was emotionally triggered and did not constitute a contraindication to surgery. Neither the cardiologist nor the neurosurgeon dealt directly with the symptom itself: What caused the head pain?
>
> The neurosurgeon then decided that her cardiac status was too questionable to risk surgery. All physicians involved in the case agreed that the actual problem of her recurrent headaches and blepharospasm was not, in fact, caused by carotid obstruction. It was anatomically and physiologically impossible. The patient, however, quite naturally believed that if surgery were performed, it would be aimed at preventing the symptoms for which she had sought medical help. Thus, she was dissatisfied and uncertain of what to do when she was discharged from the hospital without surgery.
>
> RD was subsequently seen by a general internist who emphasized that her twitching eye and headaches were a result of localized mus-

cle spasm. He taught her relaxation techniques, stressed avoidance of fatigue, and directed her attention toward assessing situations in which she found the symptoms occurring. However, she was preoccupied with the atherosclerotic lesion and decided to try chelation therapy to "dissolve" the calcium deposits.

RD later sustained a severe episode of sharp mid-chest pain after a bitter argument with her sister. She was admitted to another hospital where cardiac evaluation was again negative. While in the hospital, she developed sustained headache and blepharospasm. Repeat angiography reconfirmed her 90 percent carotid obstruction. The same neurosurgeon said he would perform the endarterectomy if she were "cardiologically stable." He seemed to want the cardiologist to veto surgery, but the cardiologist believed that, despite her recent chest pain, she was not at high risk for surgery. Subsequently, the endarterectomy was performed and she had a rocky postoperative course complicated by a left hemispheric stroke with right hemiparesis and aphasia. She continued to have blepharospasm and headache. RD was bitterly upset about this outcome and disillusioned with her doctors and with the medical care system.

This case illustrates iatrogenic suffering that has focal, behavioral, and symbolic components. **First**, the repeated invasive studies and the questionable surgical procedure caused unwarranted physical risks, were expensive, and resulted in a cerebrovascular accident. The endarterectomy presented a paradigmatic problem in contemporary medicine, a situation in which a clear disease-based indication for surgery exists, but was unrelated to the illness for which the patient sought help. **Second**, the mixed messages RD received from her physicians and their failure to address her real problems contributed to a dysfunctional behavioral pattern. The surgeon and family doctor colluded with RD in explaining her painful eye as a manifestation of carotid atherosclerosis but also avoided dealing with the issue by saying that her heart disease prohibited surgery. Other physicians said that her angina was stable and would not compromise elective surgery but that her eye symptoms resulted from muscle spasm and were unrelated to her carotid obstruction. The behavioral implications were that she assumed, more and more, an invalid role in which her life's activities were severely restricted. She also tried to resolve the problem by seeking an alternate, unorthodox approach to therapy (chelation). **Third**, the personal or symbolic implication was that she gradually became fixated on an image of herself as a "walking time bomb."

RD presented a difficult medical problem, but a major component of this difficulty arose from the "clinical distance" between her and her physicians, a distance that grew greater as the physicians came to label her as a complainer, as emotionally unstable, and as prone to dramatizing her symptoms. This "clinical distance" subtracted her as a suffering person from her diseased organs, which were the focus of her physicians' exclusive concern (Baron, 1981). Clinical situations like that of RD are usually explained by the **passive physician hypothesis:** the iatrogenic symptoms or behaviors are an inevitable result of a pattern generated by the patient. The patient's personality, coping style, or opportunity for secondary gain puts the physician in the role of ostensibly colluding, while actually just doing his or her duty as a doctor. This hypothesis would point out that RD was a "difficult patient" with a manipulative behavior pattern or had elements of hypochondriasis, features we discussed in Chapter 9. An alternate, **active physician hypothesis,** however, would recognize the symbolic and behavioral power of doctor-patient interactions. In this account, RD's physicians contributed to her suffering in a number of ways: by a failure of empathic understanding, by a lack of confidence in their own observations, and by actively helping her to "organize" the illness in a way that created the "time bomb."

The processes that lead to iatrogenic suffering are just as powerful and pervasive as their counterparts that lead to healing. In traditional societies, the healer or shaman had the power to struggle with forces causing illness, but this intimate relationship with evil was a double-edged sword. Certain shamans could turn to embrace the evil forces, thus becoming sorcerers or witches who used their esoteric knowledge to harm rather than to heal. The insight that underlies this common cultural belief is that sick people are vulnerable and the healer is powerful. Some critics of medicine hold that the imbalance of power between doctor and patient is unfortunate and remediable (Carlson, 1975; Waitzkin and Stoeckle, 1972). They argue from the premise of personal autonomy and favor a provider-consumer model of doctor-patient interaction. This position ignores the dynamic of illness. The importance of informed choice and patient education must be emphasized, but the imbalance of power between doctors and patients results not only from factors such as an information gap, a social gap, and unreformed attitudes, but also from the nature of illness itself and its power to change a person's perceptual world. Because the world of the sick is different from the world of the well, the desire to be well is often more pressing than the desire to be informed or to make choices.

The burden of suffering created by doctors and other health care personnel is partly inevitable—because we never know the consequences of all our actions—and partly avoidable. Knowledgeable integration of symbolic influences, as well as appropriate use of focal and behavioral influences, will minimize iatrogenic suffering. While medical procedures or labels are likely to have some symbolic meaning to a patient, that meaning must be ascertained on a case-by-case basis. It might be beneficial as with the upper GI x-ray series in Case 2 or harmful as with the carotid arteriography in Case 3. Sox, Margulies, and Sox reported that a group of patients, who suffered from noncardiac chest pain but who were randomly allocated to a technical evaluation including blood work and an electrocardiogram, had less short-term disability than the group not offered these tests (Sox, Margulies, and Sox, 1981). The net effect of adding these tests was more anxiety-reducing than physician-patient interaction alone in that group of patients as a whole, but if we were to study each individual case carefully, the tests may have been anxiety-provoking in some them.

THE HEALING ACT AND MEDICAL INTERVIEWING

The fact that healing involves more than a mechanistic response to the focal dimension of treatment explains why the "art of medicine" is neither a veneer of courtesy nor a collection of unsolved problems. It is, rather, the body of knowledge, skills, and judgments that grows out of the uniqueness of each doctor-patient interaction. The three-vector model of the healing act demands that **clinical judgment** not be restricted to heuristics for decision making or to mathematical models of probability. In order to manage a patient in the best way possible, the doctor must have accurate and precise information about the patient's true situation, his or her clinical reality, in order to select the right treatment. This perspective allows a broader interpretation of diagnosis and therapeutic problem-solving. It requires what the medical historian and philosopher Pedro Lain Entralgo (1969) has called an **individual diagnosis** rather than what he called the more abstract **specific diagnosis.** The latter answers the question, "What special disease is this person suffering from?" and it is our usual "medical" diagnosis. The former, however, is "the scientific understanding of what is strictly personal to the case under observation" (Lain Entralgo, 1969). It requires consideration of four major questions about the ill person. **First,** why did the illness appear when it did in the patient's life and not at another time?—the biographic occasion. **Second,** what part in the illness is played by the individuality of the patient? **Third,** how did the patient's personality or style accept or reject the illness? **Fourth,** to what extent and in what manner is the patient the creator of his or her own peculiar illness?

While we have no tests available to answer these questions with the accuracy or precision of a blood creatinine determination, they can still be approached systematically through good medical interviewing techniques. Admittedly, we lack empirical data about the effects of such an "individual" approach to diagnosis and treatment. It will be difficult to design studies to demonstrate effectiveness; yet several commentators have given us testable approaches or constructs to address individuality in healing. They include an approach to eliciting the patient's model of clinical reality (Kleinman, Eisenberg, and Good, 1978), the health belief model (Becker and Marmon, 1975), cognitive approaches to improving doctor-patient communication (Ley, 1976), the patient evaluation grid (Leigh and Reiser, 1980), the "actual reason for coming" versus the "ostensible reason for coming" (Bass and Cohen, 1982), and new typologies of illness (Barondess, 1983). Norman Cousins called on physicians to employ artistry to potentiate and motivate their patients—a behavioral influence (Cousins, 1982); but through clinical judgment they should also employ artistry to select the correct individual diagnosis and treatment—focal and symbolic influences.

The three-vector model should also enhance your respect for symptoms, as well as your interest in the physiology of these symptoms. Physicians know a great deal about human physiology but often relatively little about the specific physiology of a symptom. If symptoms are only fellow-travelers, bearing some direct necessary relationship to an underlying disease, treatment of symptoms is only a secondary issue at best. It has little intrinsic interest. But if symptoms are the net effect both of disease and of multiple levels of meaning, all of which is manifest as physiologic change, then a therapeutic focus on symptoms becomes important. It is possible that controlling a symptom, as in our Case 1, may have important healing effects that go beyond the symptom itself. It is possible that an aggressive approach to controlling RD's symptom in Case 3 would have led to a vastly different outcome of her problem. We believe that physicians should teach people about why their bodies have a symptom and what they can do about it; this teaching can and should begin during the initial patient interview.

This book addresses the first step in the clinical art: communication between doctor and patient. The "subjective" data of symptoms and suffering are at the core of medical practice and can be made more "objective" through skillful, systematic attention. We have described and illustrated medical history taking that will allow you to begin making both appropriate **specific diagnoses** of disease and careful **individual diagnoses** of illness. This is the first step on the road to enhancing behavioral and symbolic influences in all your interactions with patients, while minimizing iatrogenic suffering.

References/Bibliography

Books

AMERICAN PSYCHIATRIC ASSOCIATION: *Diagnostic and Statistical Manual of Mental Disorders.* ed 3. Washington, DC, 1980.

BALINT, M: *The Doctor, His Patient and the Illness* (rev American ed). International Universities Press, New York, 1972.

CARLSON, RJ: *The End of Medicine.* John Wiley & Sons, New York, 1975.

CARROLL, LEWIS: *The Annotated Alice: Alice's Adventures in Wonderland and Through the Looking Glass.* GARDNER, MARTIN (ED). Clarkson N. Potter, New York, 1960, p 323.

CASSELL, EJ: *The Healer's Art.* JB Lippincott, Philadelphia and New York, 1976.

CASSELL, EJ: *Talking With Patients.* Vol 1: Theory of Doctor-Patient Communication. Vol 2: Clinical Technique. MIT Press, Cambridge, MA, 1985.

CUTLER, P: *Problem Solving in Clinical Medicine.* Williams & Wilkins, Baltimore, 1979.

DOYLE, A. CONAN: *Adventures of Sherlock Holmes.* Harper & Row, New York, 1966, p 54.

ELSTEIN, AS, SCHULMAN, LS, AND SPRAFKA, SA: *Medical Problem Solving: An Analysis of Clinical Reasoning.* Harvard University Press, Cambridge, MA, 1978.

FEINSTEIN, A: *Clinical Judgment.* Williams & Wilkins, Baltimore, 1967.

GRECO, RS AND PITTENGER, RA: *One Man's Practice.* Tavestock Publications, JB Lippincott, Philadelphia, 1966.

IVEY, AE AND AUTHIER, J: *Microcounselling.* Charles C Thomas, Springfield, IL, 1978.

KIMBALL, CP: *The Biopsychosocial Approach to the Patient.* Williams & Wilkins, Baltimore, 1981.

KRAYTMAN, M: *The Complete Medical History.* McGraw-Hill, New York, 1979.

LAIN ENTRALGO, P: *Doctor and Patient.* World University Library, McGraw-Hill, New York, 1969, pp 199–205.

LIDZ, CW, ROTH, LH, ZERUBAVEL, E, ET AL: *Informed Consent: A Study of Psychiatric Decision-Making.* Gurlford Press, New York, 1983.

LEIGH, H AND REISER, MF: *The Patient. Biological, Psychological and Social Dimensions of Medical Practice.* Plenum Medical Books, New York, 1980.

PENDLETON, D AND HASLER, J (EDS): *Doctor-Patient Communication.* Academic Press, New York, 1983.

RAKEL, RE: *Principles of Family Medicine.* WB Saunders, Philadelphia, 1977.

REILLY, BM: *Practical Strategies in Outpatient Medicine.* WB Saunders, Philadelphia, 1984.

REISER, DE AND SCHRODER, AK: *Patient Interviewing: The Human Dimension.* Williams & Wilkins, Baltimore, 1980.

ROGERS, C: *On Becoming a Person.* Houghton Mifflin, Boston, 1961.

RUSSEL, BERTRAND: *The Problems of Philosophy.* Oxford University Press, London, 1912.

SACKETT, DL AND HAYNES, RB: *Compliance with Therapeutic Regimens.* Johns Hopkins University Press, Baltimore, 1976.

SANDNER, D: *Navajo Symbols of Healing.* Harcourt Brace Jovanovich, New York, 1979, p 11.

TOLSTOY, LEO: *The Death of Ivan Ilych.* Signet Classics, New York, 1960, p 121.

Journal Articles and Book Chapters

AYER, AJ: *The Problem of Knowledge.* Chapter 4. St. Martin's Press, New York, 1956.

BARON, RJ: *Bridging clinical distance: An empathic rediscovery of the known.* J Med Philosophy 6:5, 1981.

BARONDESS, JA: *The clinical transaction: Themes and descants.* Perspect Biol Med 27:25, 1983.

BASS, LW AND COHEN, RL: *Ostensible versus actual reasons for seeking pediatric attention: Another look at the parental ticket of admission.* Pediatrics 70:870, 1982.

BECKER, MH AND MAIMAN, LA: *Sociobehavioral determinants of compliance with health and medical care recommendations.* Med Care 13:10, 1975.

BEECHER, HK: *The powerful placebo.* JAMA 159:1602, 1955.

BERNARDE, MA AND MAYERSON, EW: *Patient-physician negotiation.* JAMA 239:1413, 1978.

BERTAKIS, KD: *From physician to patient: A method for increasing patient retention and satisfaction.* J Fam Pract 5:217, 1977.

BRODY, DS: *The patient's role in clinical decision-making.* Ann Int Med 93:718, 1980.

BRODY, H: *The lie that heals: The ethics of giving placebos.* Ann Int Med 97:112, 1982.

COULEHAN, JL: *Adjustment, the hands and healing.* Culture, Medicine and Psychiatry (in press, 1985).

COULEHAN, JL: *Ascorbic acid and the common cold. Reviewing the evidence.* Postgrad Med 66:153, 1979.

COULEHAN, JL: *Dissecting the clinical art.* The Pharos 47(4):21, 1984.

COULEHAN, JL: *The treatment act: A model with focal, behavioral and symbolic dimensions.* Marriage and Family Review (in press).

COULEHAN, JL AND BLOCK, M: *Creating the healing connection.* In LAZES, P: *Handbook of Health Education,* ed 2. Aspen Press, 1986.

COUSINS, N: *Physician as communicator.* JAMA 248:587, 1982.

DEWEY, JOHN: *Propositions, Warranted Assertibility, and Truth.* In NAGEL, E AND BRANDT, R: *Meaning and Knowledge: Systematic Readings in Epistomology.* Harcourt, Brace, & World, New York, 1965, p 154.

DROSSMAN, DA: *The problem patient. Evaluation and care of medical patients with psychosocial disturbances.* Ann Int Med 88:366, 1978.

EGBERT, LD, BATTIT, GE, WELCH, CE, ET AL: *Reduction of postoperative pain by encouragement and instruction of patients.* N Engl J Med 270:825, 1964.

EISENBERG, L: *What makes persons "patients" and patients "well"?* Am J Med 69:277, 1980.

EISENBERG, L AND KLEINMAN, A: *Clinical social science.* In EISENBERG, L AND KLEINMAN, A (EDS): *The Relevance of Social Science for Medicine.* D Reidel Publishing, Dordrecht, Netherlands, 1980.

ENGEL, GL: *The care of the patient: Art or science?* Johns Hopkins Med J 140:222, 1977.

ERAKER, SA AND POLITSER, P: *How decisions are reached: Physician and patient.* Ann Int Med 97:262, 1982.

FEINSTEIN, AR: *An additional basic science for clinical medicine: IV the development of clinometrics.* Ann Int Med 99:843, 1983.

FRANK, JD: *The faith that heals.* Johns Hopkins Med J 137:127, 1975.

GOLDMAN, RH AND PETERS, JM: *The occupational and environmental health history.* JAMA 246:2831, 1981.

GOODWIN, JS, GOODWIN, JM, AND VOGEL, AV: *Knowledge and use of placebos by house officers and nurses.* Ann Int Med 91:106, 1979.

GREY, G AND FLYNN, P: *A survey of placebo use in a general hospital.* Gen Hosp Psychiatry 3:199, 1981.

GROVES, JE: *Taking care of the hateful patient.* N Engl J Med 398:883, 1978.

GUTHEIL, TG, BURSZTAJN, H, AND BRODSKY, A: *Malpractice prevention through the sharing of uncertainty. Informed consent and the therapeutic alliance.* N Engl J Med 311:49, 1984.

HEATON, PB: *Negotiation as an integral part of the physician's clinical reasoning.* J Fam Pract 13:845, 1981.

HOUSTON, WR: *The doctor himself as therapeutic agent.* Ann Int Med 11:1416, 1938.

KAHANA, RJ AND BIBRING, GL: *Personality Types in Medical Management.* In ZINBERG, NE (ED): *Psychiatry and Medical Practice in a General Hospital.* International Universities Press, New York, 1964, pp 108–123.

KIMBALL, CP: *Techniques of interviewing. Interviewing and the meaning of the symptom.* Ann Intern Med 71:147, 1969.

KLEINMAN, A, EISENBERG, L, AND GOOD, B: *Culture, illness and care, clinical lessons from anthropological and cross-cultural research.* Ann Int Med 88:251, 1978.

LASAGNA, L, MOSTELLER, F, VON FELSINGER, JM, ET AL: *A study of the placebo response.* Am J Med 16:770, 1954.

LEY, P: *Satisfaction, compliance and communication.* Br J Clin Psychol 21:241, 1982.

LEY, P: *Toward better doctor-patient communication. Contributions from social and experimental psychology.* In BENNETT, AE (ED): *Communication Between Doctors and Patients.* Oxford University Press, Oxford, Nuffield Provincial Hospitals Trust, 1976, pp 77–98.

LIPOWSKI, ZJ: *Physical illness, the individual and the coping process.* Psychiatry Med 1:91, 1970.

MOERTL, CG, ET AL: *Who responds to sugar pills?* Mayo Clin Proc 5:96, 1976.

MUMFORD, E, SCHLESINGER, HJ, AND GLASS, GV: *The effects of psychological intervention on recovery from surgery and heart attacks: An analysis of the literature.* Am J Pub Health 72:141, 1982.

PELLEGRINO, ED: *The healing relationship: The architectonics of clinical medicine.* In SHELP, E (ED): *The Clinical Encounter.* D Reidel Publishing, Dordrecht, Netherlands, 1983, pp 153–172.

PENICK, SB AND HINKLE, LE: *The effect of expectation on response to phenmetrazine.* Psychosom Med 26:369, 1964.

PLATO: *The Laws.* In HAMILTON, E AND CAIRNS, H (EDS): *The Collected Dialogues of Plato.* Bollingen Foundation, New York, 1961.

PLATT, FW AND MCMATH, JC: *Clinical hypocompetence: The interview.* Ann Int Med 91:898, 1979.

ROE, W: *"Science" in the practice of medicine: Its limitations and dangers.* Perspect Biol Med 27:386, 1984.

SARLES, H, CAMATTE, R, SAHEL, J, ET AL: *A study of the variations in the response regarding duodenal ulcer when treated with placebo.* Digestion 16:289, 1977.

SHAKESPEARE, WILLIAM: *The Tragedie of Romeo and Juliet.* In *Complete Works of William Shakespeare.* Doubleday, New York, 1946.

SHAPIRO, AK: *The placebo response.* In HOWELLS, JG (ED): *Modern Perspectives in World Psychiatry,* Vol. 2. Oliver and Boyd, Edinburgh, 1971.

SIEGLER, M: *The physician-patient accommodation. A central event in clinical medicine.* Arch Intern Med 142:1899, 1982.

SNOW, LF: *Folk medical beliefs and their implications for care of patients.* Ann Int Med 81:82, 1974.

Sox, HC, Margulies, I, and Sox, CH: *Psychologically mediated effects of diagnostic tests.* Ann Int Med 95:680, 1981.

Talbot, NA: *The position of the Christian Science Church.* N Engl J Med 309:1641, 1983.

Thompson, R: *Side effects and placebo administration.* Br J Psychiatry 140:64, 1982.

Tversky, A and Kahneman, D: *Judgment under uncertainty: Heuristics and biases.* Science 185:1124, 1974.

Uzzell, D: *Susto revisited: Illness as strategic role.* In Landy, D (ED): *Culture, Disease and Healing.* Macmillan, New York, 1978.

Waitzkin, H and Stoeckle, JD: *The communication of information about illness. Clinical, sociological, and methodological considerations.* Adv Psychosom Med 8:180, 1972.

Weiner, S and Nathanson, M: *Physical examination. Frequently observed errors.* JAMA 236:852, 1976.

Wilde, Oscar: *The Critic as Artist: With Some Remarks upon the Importance of Discussing Everything.* A Dialogue, Part II. In Wilde, Oscar: *Selected Writings.* Oxford University Press, London, 1961, p 99.

Wolraich, ML, Albanese, M, Reiter-Thayer, S, et al: *Factors Affecting Physician Communication and Parent-Physician Dialogues.* J Med Education 57:621–625, 1982.

Wright, AD, Green, ID, Fleetwood-Walker, DM, et al: *Patterns of acquisition of interview skills by medical students.* Lancet 1:964, 1980.

Some Words to Describe Feelings

Abandoned	Bitter	Creative
Adamant	Blamed	Cruel
Afraid	Blissful	Crummy
Aggravated	Blocked	Crushed
Agitated	Blue	Curious
Agony	Bold	
Alert	Bored	Deceitful
Alienated	Bothered	Deceived
Alive	Brave	Defeated
Alone	Bugged	Defiant
Amazed	Burdened	Degraded
Ambiguous		Dejected
Ambivalent	Callous	Delerious
Amused	Calm	Delighted
Angry	Capable	Depressed
Annoyed	Captivated	Despair
Anxious	Cautious	Destructive
Apathetic	Challenged	Determined
Appalled	Charmed	Devastated
Apprehensive	Cheated	Different
Ashamed	Cheerful	Diffident
Assured	Childish	Dirty
Astounded	Clever	Disappointed
Astonished	Combative	Discontented
At ease	Comfortable	Discouraged
Awed	Committed	Disgusted
Awkward	Compassionate	Disoriented
	Concerned	Dissatisfied
Backward	Condemned	Distracted
Bad	Confident	Distraught
Bashful	Conflicted	Distressed
Beligerent	Confused	Distrustful
Belittled	Consumed	Disturbed
Betrayed	Contented	Dominated
Bewildered	Contrite	Doubtful
Bitchy	Controlled	Down

Downtrodden
Drained
Driven
Dubious
Dumb

Eager
Ecstatic
Edgy
Elated
Embarrassed
Empty
Enchanted
Encouraged
Energetic
Enervated
Engrossed
Engulfed
Enlightened
Enraged
Enthusiastic
Envious
Euphoric
Evil
Exasperated
Excited
Exhausted

Fantastic
Fawning
Fearful
Flustered
Foolish
Forgotten
Forlorn
Fragmented
Frantic
Frenzied
Fretful
Friendly
Frightened
Frustrated
Funny
Furious
Fury

Gay
Glad
Gloomy
Glum
Good
Grateful
Gratified

Great
Grief
Groovy
Grouchy
Guilty
Gullible

Happy
Hassled
Hateful
Helpful
Helpless
Hesitant
High
Hopeful
Hopeless
Horrible
Horrified
Hostile
Hurt
Hysterical

Ignorant
Ignored
Impatient
Impulsive
Important
Inadequate
Incapable
Incompetent
Independent
Indifferent
Inferior
Infuriated
Insecure
Insensitive
Inspired
Interested
Intimidated
Involved
Irritated
Isolated

Jealous
Jittery
Joyful
Jubilant
Jumpy

Laconic
Lazy
Left out
Let down

Lethargic
Licentious
Light hearted
Listless
Lonely
Longing
Loved
Loving
Low

Mad
Manipulated
Marvelous
Maudlin
Mean
Meek
Melancholy
Mellow
Miserable
Misunderstood
Mixed up
Modest
Morose
Mystified

Needed
Negative
Neglected
Nervous
Nice
Numb
Nutty

Obnoxious
Obsessed
Odd
Oppressed
Outraged
Overwhelmed

Pain
Pained
Panicked
Patient
Peaceful
Perplexed
Persecuted
Perturbed
Petrified
Phony
Picked on
Pity
Pleasant

Pleased
Positive
Pressured
Preoccupied
Proud
Pushed
Put down
Put upon
Puzzled

Quarrelsome
Queer
Quiet

Rage
Refreshed
Regretful
Rejected
Rejuvenated
Relaxed
Relieved
Remorseful
Renewed
Resentful
Resigned
Restless
Rewarded
Righteous
Rotten

Sad
Safe
Satisfied
Scared
Scattered
Screwed up
Secure
Selfish
Sensitive
Sensuous
Serious

Shattered
Shocked
Shy
Sick
Silly
Skeptical
Smothered
Sober
Solemn
Sophisticated
Sorrowful
Sorry
Spiteful
Strange
Strong
Stubborn
Stunned
Stupefied
Stupid
Successful
Suffering
Superfluous
Superior
Sure
Surprised
Suspicious
Sympathetic

Tense
Tentative
Tenuous
Terrible
Testy
Threatened
Thwarted
Tired
Tormented
Torn
Tranquil
Trapped
Tremendous

Troubled
Turned on (off)
Terrific
Terrified

Ugly
Unafraid
Uncertain
Uncomfortable
Uneasy
Unfortunate
Unhappy
Unimportant
Uninvolved
Unlucky
Unpleasant
Unsettled
Unwanted
Upset
Uptight
Useful
Useless

Vehement
Violent
Vital
Vivacious
Vulnerable

Warm
Weak
Wary
Weepy
Whimsical
Whole
Wicked
Wonderful
Worried
Worthless
Worthwhile

An Annotated Medical Interview

This is a slightly altered typescript (to protect the patient's privacy) taken from a real interview of a new patient by a medical intern. It is not presented as an ideal or exhaustive medical history but simply as a good example of an empathic and careful interview. The patient comes in to the clinic for a "check-up."

Typescript	Comments
Dr: I guess the best place to start is to ask you what brings you here today.	Opening.
Pt: Well, I haven't had a physical really since five years ago, since my son was born.	
Dr: I am going to be writing some things down on paper here, okay? Is there any particular reason why you chose now to come in?	Acknowledges note taking. Open-ended question. Probe for iatrotropic stimulus.
Pt: I figured I kept putting it off and putting it off. I'd make appointments and put them off. There was no particular reason. I just felt as though it was time, I suppose.	
Dr: Nothing is bothering you at this point?	
Pt: No, it's just that I am overweight, that's all. I go up and down, up and down.	
Dr: So that was your major concern, the weight problem?	Summary statement. Interchangeable response.
Pt: Yeah.	
Dr: Can you tell me about that?	Open-ended question.
Pt: Well, I've always been big. All the women in my family are big. It's never slowed me down or anything, but I would like to just like firm up, maybe my thighs and my stomach. From after having children I don't know, they say everything takes time, you don't put it on right away, but I guess I'm impatient.	

204

Dr:	How much do you weigh right now?	The doctor inquires in detail about the symptom—what, how much, when, why?—developing accuracy and precision.
Pt:	I don't basically know. Last time I weighed myself I weighed 200 pounds and that was like about two months ago.	
Dr:	Say a year ago, what did you weigh?	
Pt:	A year ago I weighed about 230 pounds.	
Dr:	230 pounds? So you have actually lost 30 pounds between then and now?	The doctor checks back with patient, comfirming data.
Pt:	Yes.	
Dr:	Have you been on a diet?	
Pt:	No.	
Dr:	How have you lost the weight?	
Pt:	I don't know. In the last, I'd say the last 6 months or so to a year, I've been getting to the point I'd go all day without eating. I'm real active. I'm very active.	
Dr:	Can you tell me about the activity?	Open-ended question with topic specified.
Pt:	Well, I do a lot of tennis. I have dance class. It seems like I don't want to stop to fix nothing when I'm working in the house. I won't stop to fix nothing to eat. I'll just keep on going.	
Dr:	Is that a conscious effort on your part, to try to lose weight?	
Pt:	I don't know if it's subconscious or conscious. I really never set down and thought about it.	
Dr:	Was that something you're attempting to do? That's one of your goals?	
Pt:	Yeah, something like that.	
Dr:	How many children did you say you had?	A series of closed questions.
Pt:	Four.	
Dr:	Before you had your first child, how much did you weigh?	
Pt:	I weighed about 140 pounds.	
Dr:	And how old were you then?	
Pt:	I was 18.	
Dr:	How many years ago was that?	
Pt:	Thirteen years ago.	
Dr:	When would you say that you had gained the majority of weight between then and now?	
Pt:	When I had my second child.	
Dr:	How much did you weigh at that times, before the second child?	
Pt:	Before? Before my second child, I weighed around 150 to 160.	
Dr:	What do you think it was between then and now that's made you gain the weight?	

Pt:	Nerves made me do a lot of eating. Then a lot of marital problems.	
Dr:	Do you want to discuss that a little bit more?	Open-ended question, leading to further exploration of possible emotional etiologies for weight change.
Pt:	Oh, it was just a thing, me and my husband were—just like any other marriage I guess—good times, bad times—but more bad times than good. I had gotten to the point that I felt as though, I got all these children, what am I worth? You know, that kind of depressed me a little bit and I started gaining all that weight. After I had my last child I don't know, something just hit me, and I came up out of that.	
Dr:	When was that?	
Pt:	Five years ago.	
Dr:	So, how would you describe your general mood now?	Open-ended question, topic specified.
Pt:	Fine.	
Dr:	You don't feel anything is wrong?	
Pt:	No. I very seldom—last time I got depressed was one day about two months ago 'cause there wasn't no jobs and that's about it. But depression, I can't remember at all when I last felt depression. I feel good about myself, good about my surroundings, 'cause you know you are only doing the best you can.	
Dr:	What do you think has brought about that change?	
Pt:	I don't know what it was really. I really don't. Well, after me and my husband had separated, I started feeling good about myself because for one, I got to the point, well, the children have to depend on me now, because I was doing a lot of depending on him.	
Dr:	When exactly was that?	
Pt:	That was about three years ago.	
Dr:	So since then you have generally felt better about yourself.	A summarization of the patient's statement.
Pt:	Yeah.	
Dr:	Can you describe your eating habits over the past several years?	
Pt:	Okay, well, I eat breakfast. I eat sometimes a large breakfast and during the mid-day I'll drink tea, eat some fruit, drink milk. I drink a lot of milk. I love milk. I might sit down and eat dinner about—lunch, I don't even worry about lunch 'cause I never see it. I eat dinner about 6 or 7 o'clock in the evening. In the last couple months I stopped	

snacking on a lot of sweets. Before I used to crave them at a certain period of the time, mostly when it was my menstrual period, I'd crave a lot of sweets. Lately I just don't even care for sweets too much. But I still drink a lot of milk, as long as it's cold, I'll drink a lot of milk.

Dr: So you eat basically two meals a day.

> Checking back about important data.

Pt: Yeah, sometimes one.

Dr: And you don't do much snacking between meals.

Pt: No.

Dr: Now besides this weight problem, which seems to be improving, do you have any other complaints?

> The doctor asks about other current problems—perhaps an iatrotropic stimulus as yet unmentioned.

Pt: None whatsoever.

Dr: None whatsoever?

> With a mild confrontation the doctor elicits a new concern—edema.

Pt: Yeah—now, weird as it might sound, now my ankles—on my right leg, my ankle will not swell up, but my left leg swells up. And I was taking water pills there for awhile from a doctor.

Dr: How long has this been going on?

> Beginning of questions defining and categorizing causes of edema.

Pt: I'd say for three months.

Dr: When is the ankle swelling worse? Is it during the morning when you wake up?

Pt: No, during the evening.

Dr: As the day wears on?

Pt: Yeah, as the day wears on.

Dr: When you wake up in the morning, are they decreased?

Pt: Yes.

Dr: How many pillows do you sleep on?

Pt: One.

Dr: Do you ever wake up in the middle of the night gasping for air?

Pt: No.

Dr: How many times do you go the bathroom at night?

Pt: About once.

Dr: And that's your only other major complaint at this time?

Pt: Yes.

Dr: Have you had any change in bowel habits?

> Beginning of some ROS-type questions probing specifically for symptoms of thyroid disease.

Pt: No.

Dr: Constipation? Diarrhea?

Pt:	No.	
Dr:	Change in your voice?	
Pt:	Yeah, my voice has gotten heavier.	
Dr:	How long has that gone on?	
Pt:	I'd say in the about the last year and a half.	
Dr:	Any change in your skin or your hair?	An open-ended question, which requires additional specification for this patient.
Pt:	My hair has gotten longer.	
Dr:	Besides longer, the quality of your skin or your hair?	
Pt:	My skin is getting—I don't know—a couple of years ago I just looked like I was older and maybe I just started taking better care of myself.	
Dr:	Okay, but you wouldn't say that there was any thinning or thickening of your skin or anything like that?	
Pt:	No.	
Dr:	Do you ever feel hot in a room where everyone else is cold or cold whenever everyone else is hot?	
Pt:	I can't stand heat. I cannot stand heat at all. Summertime I stay in the house until the evenings. I've always been like that. Cold weather I love.	
Dr:	Do you have any allergies?	Beginning of past medical history.
Pt:	I have bronchitis.	
Dr:	But any drug allergies that you are aware of?	
Pt:	No.	
Dr:	Any medications that you are taking?	
Pt:	No. I'm allergic to penicillin.	
Dr.:	Ok, you are allergic to penicillin.	
Pt:	Yeah.	
Dr:	What does penicillin do to you?	Note the clarification—what does "allergy" mean?
Pt:	I broke out in hives.	
Dr:	Do you know of any medical problems that you have had in the past? Any high blood pressure?	
Pt:	No. I have low blood. I'm anemic.	
Dr:	You're anemic?	
Pt:	Yes.	
Dr:	How long have you had the anemia?	
Pt:	Since I've had my first child.	
Dr:	Have you taken anything for it?	
Pt:	I used to take iron pills there for awhile. That was about 10 years ago, then I just stopped because they made me feel tired.	
Dr:	How's your pep and energy been?	
Pt:	Fine.	
Dr:	Any shortness of breath?	

Pt: No.
Dr: Any problems with your heart?
Pt: No.
Dr: Heart attacks?
Pt: No.
Dr: Heart murmurs?
Pt: No.
Dr: Rheumatic heart disease?
Pt: No.
Dr: Have you ever had any strokes?
Pt: No.
Dr: Problems with your lungs?
Pt: No.
Dr: Asthma? Tuberculosis? Bronchitis?
Pt: Bronchitis.
Dr: How does that show itself?

The doctor asks for primary observations; does not accept interpretation.

Pt: Last time I had—it showed itself bad—it was like 10 years ago and I was in the hospital for that.
Dr: Do you have any cough now?
Pt: Yeah, 'cause I smoke.
Dr: Do you cough up any sputum?
Pt: Yeah.
Dr: How much sputum?
Pt: Not very much.
Dr: What would you think? More than a shot glass?
Pt: No.
Dr: And what does it look like, the sputum?
Pt: It's white.
Dr: Any other problems? Stomach ulcers?
Pt: No.
Dr: Seizures?
Pt: No.
Dr: Problems with your kidneys or liver?
Pt: No.
Dr: Any operations in the past?
Pt: I had my tubes tied five years ago.
Dr: Was that with your last child?
Pt: Yes.
Dr: Did you make that decision?
Pt: Yes.
Dr: How do you feel about that decision?

The doctor elicits the patient's feelings about a potentially sensitive issue (which might bear upon her weight problem).

Pt: At that time I felt good. Then a couple years ago I met this friend and I felt bad about it because I wanted to have another child. And I snapped out of that real quick.
Dr: But you've gotten over that?

Pt:	Yes.
Dr:	Any other operations that you remember?
Pt:	No.
Dr:	Tonsils?
Pt:	No.
Dr:	Appendix? Gallbladder?
Pt:	No.
Dr:	So you have five children now?

Beginning of the "social history," but notice how much you already know about this person from the manner in which the present illness inquiry is conducted.

Pt:	Four.
Dr:	Four children.
Pt:	Yes.
Dr:	And are they all living at home with you?
Pt:	Yes.
Dr:	What are their ages?
Pt:	13, 11, 8, 5.
Dr:	Are they all in good health?
Pt:	Yes.
Dr:	Are you fortunate enough to have a job right now?

Notice how well this question is put *(respect)*.

Pt:	No, not right now.
Dr:	What type of work did you do in the past?
Pt:	I've done various things. I drove a bus, did maintenance work, cashier in a store.
Dr:	How long have you been unemployed?
Pt:	For about two months now.
Dr:	Any prospects?
Pt:	No, just a lot of applications in. That's about it.
Dr:	How does that feel? You must be upset.

Attempt at interchangeable response.

Pt:	Not really. Something will come up. Something's bound to come up.
Dr:	So you are optimistic?

Successful interchangeable response.

Pt:	Yeah.
Dr:	You said you smoked cigarettes. How much do you smoke?

Transition to new topic.

Pt:	I smoke—a pack will last me about 2 days.
Dr:	How long have you smoked?
Pt:	I've been smoking since I was 16.
Dr:	Right now, you're 31?
Pt:	Right, I'll be 32 in July.
Dr:	Drink any alcohol?
Pt:	No.
Dr:	Have you ever?
Pt:	Yes, I stopped drinking when I was 18.
Dr:	Why was that?
Pt:	I was pregnant with my first child.
Dr:	Do you use any other type of drugs?

Pt: No.
Dr: Are your parents living?

Beginning of family health history.

Pt: My mother is.
Dr: How old is she?
Pt: 60.
Dr: And your father?
Pt: He's deceased.
Dr: How old was he when he passed away?
Pt: I was 15 years old.
Dr: You can just take a guess.
Pt: I'd say in his 40s I guess.
Dr: Do you know how he passed away?
Pt: He had a heart attack.
Dr: Did he have any diabetes or high blood pressure?
Pt: He had high blood.
Dr: Any strokes?
Pt: No.
Dr: How about your mother? How's her health?
Pt: Fine. She has a—I forget what they call it but it's connected with a hernia.
Dr: Do you have brothers and sisters?
Pt: Yes, one brother and one sister.
Dr: How's their health?
Pt: Fine.
Dr: Any brothers or sisters passed away?
Pt: No.
Dr: Are there any diseases or illnesses that run in your family?
Pt: No.
Dr: Heart conditions? High blood pressure? Diabetes?
Pt: Yeah, my uncle had—he was a diabetic.
Dr: I'm just going to run through a bunch of questions now. Have you had any headaches recently?

Transition and beginning of formal review of systems.

Pt: No.
Dr: Blurred or double vision?
Pt: In one eye. This one jumps. It's the left one. That's been about 3 months now.
Dr: What do you mean by jumps?

Attempt at establishing precise meaning.

Pt: It gets to quivering. I don't know whether it's nerves. I used to say something's going to happen.
Dr: Any blind spots in your eyes?
Pt: No.
Dr: Do you see double out of that eye?
Pt: No. Once in awhile when I come in from a different room area. Like this one will kind of dart and then it will clear up and my vision gets together.

Dr: Any difficulty hearing?
Pt: No.
Dr: Any bleeding through your nose, mouth, lips, and gums? Difficulty swallowing?
Pt: No.
Dr: Shortness of breath or wheezing?
Pt: Wheezing.
Dr: When do you have the wheezing?
Pt: At night when I sleep.
Dr: Do you take anything for that?
Pt: No, not really.
Dr: Do you get up, or does it just go away?
Pt: Sometimes I'll get up and drink some water and that's it.
Dr: How often do you get that?
Pt: Every night during the night.
Dr: Coughing any blood up at all?
Pt: No.
Dr: Any fever, chills, or sweats?
Pt: No.
Dr: Belly pain?
Pt: No.
Dr: Lumps or bumps anywhere in your breasts or under your arms?
Pt: No.
(Interruption at door.)
Dr: What was I asking you, about belly pains?
Pt: Yes.
Dr: No belly pains?
Pt: No.
Dr: Diarrhea or constipation?
Pt: No.
Dr: Any blood in your stools?
Pt: No.
Dr: Any swelling of any of your joints or joint pains?
Pt: Just my ankles.
Dr: Okay, we already talked about that. Any rash anywhere on your body?
Pt: No.
Dr: I think that's about all the questions. Do you have any questions for me? Is there anything else?   Inviting the patient to have the last word.
Pt: No.
Dr: I think we have covered mostly everything.   Closing.

Index

Numbers in *italics* indicate figures; numbers followed by a "t" indicate tables.

medical interview and, 113

NEGOTIATION, compliance and, 168–174
Nonverbal communication
  as fundamental skill, 33–35
  gestures, 35–37

OBJECTIVITY, of history taking, 5–7
  interpretation versus, 7–9
Observer bias(es), 114
Occam's razor, as psychologic bias in clinical judgment, 108t, 110–111
Open-ended (or nondirective) questions, to elicit present illness in medical history, 44, 45–46, 47t
Orderly, controlled patient, 135–136. See also Difficult interview, patient personality styles in

PARALINGUISTICS, nonverbal communication and, 37
Passive physician hypothesis, 194
Past medical history (PMH), 56–61, 57t
Patient(s)
  in difficult interviews
    types of
      rambling, 115t, 119–120
      reticent, 115t, 117–119
      vague, 115t, 120–122
    personality styles of, 133–134
      dependent, demanding, 134–135
      dramatizing, manipulative, 137
      guarded, paranoid, 139
      long-suffering, masochistic, 137–139
      orderly, controlled, 135–136
      superior, 139–140
Patient interview(s), 3. See also Medical interview(s)
Patient profile(s), in medical history, 74–77
  cigarette, alcohol, and illicit drug use, 81
  demographics, 77
  diet, 79
  family, 77
  impact of illness, 80
  lifestyle, 77–79
  marital and/or significant relationships, 80–81
  occupation, 77–78t
  support system, 80
Personality, patient, styles of, 133–134
  dependent, demanding, 134–135
  dramatizing, manipulative, 137
  guarded, paranoid, 139

long-suffering, masochistic, 137–139
  orderly, controlled, 135–136
  superior, 139–140
Physical examination(s)
  conversation during, 87–91
  touching and, 94–95
  transition from medical history to, 85–86
  uses of, 91–94, 92t
Physiology, "folk," 162–163
Pill(s), sugar, placebo effect, 176–178
Placebo(s), 175
Placebo effect(s), 175–176
  as symbolic influences, 176
    clinical trials, 179–180
    doctor-patient interaction, 182–185
    iatroplacebogenesis and, 176
    sugar pills, 176–178
    unorthodox healing, 180–182
  iatroplacebogenesis and, 176
Planning, reasoned, clinical judgment in medical interview and, 113
PMH. See Past medical history (PMH)
"Poor historian," 1–4
Precision
  clinical judgment in medical interview and, 112
  in history taking, 9–11
Privacy, sense of, setting of medical history and, 39
Probability
  clinical judgment in medical interview and, 107–108, 112
  biases in, 108
  hypotheses and, 107–108
  revision of, clinical judgment in medical interview and, 113
Probability testing
  clinical judgment in medical interview and, 107–108
Problem(s), in difficult interview
  personality styles and feelings, 133–134
  process, 115, 115t
    style impairments, 115t, 117
      rambling patient, 115t, 119–120
      reticent patient, 115t, 117–119
      vague patient, 115t, 120–122
    storytelling, 122–123
    technical impairments, 115t, 116–117
  technical. See Problem(s), process
  topical, 115t, 116, 123
    drug and alcohol use, 123–125
    positive ROS, 131–132
    reliability and, 125–126